OCCUPATIONAL THERAPY

A Guide for Prospective Students,
Consumers, and Advocates

OCCUPATIONAL THERAPY

A Guide for Prospective Students, Consumers, and Advocates

Franklin Stein, PhD, OTR/L, FAOTA

Kathlyn L. Reed, PhD, OTR, FAOTA, MLIS

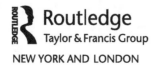

Routledge
Taylor & Francis Group

NEW YORK AND LONDON

First published 2021 by SLACK Incorporated

Published 2024 by Routledge
605 Third Avenue, New York, NY 10158

and by Routledge
4 Park Square, Milton Park, Abingdon, Oxon, OX14 4RN

Routledge is an imprint of the Taylor & Francis Group, an informa business

Library of Congress Cataloging-in-Publication Data

Names: Stein, Franklin, author. | Reed, Kathlyn L., author.
Title: Occupational therapy : a guide for prospective students, consumers, and advocates / Franklin Stein, Kathlyn L. Reed.
Description: Thorofare, NJ : SLACK Incorporated, [2021] | Includes bibliographical references and index.
Identifiers: LCCN 2020041772 (print) | ISBN 9781630918163 (paperback)
Subjects: MESH: Occupational Therapy | Vocational Guidance
Classification: LCC RM735.3 (print) | NLM WB 555 |
  DDC 615.8/515--dc23
LC record available at https://lccn.loc.gov/2020041772

Cover Artist: Katherine Christie

ISBN: 9781630918163 (pbk)
ISBN: 9781003526575 (ebk)

DOI: 10.4324/9781003526575

DEDICATION

We dedicate this book to the hundreds of thousands of occupational therapists throughout the world who strive to help people with physical and psychological disabilities of all ages to become as independent as possible in their daily living activities.

CONTENTS

PHOTO CREDIT

Chapter 1 opening photo (p. 1) from Halfpoint via Shutterstock.

Chapter 2 opening photo (p. 7) reprinted with permission from 1990 American Occupational Therapy Association (AOTA) Calendar.

Chapter 3 opening photo (p. 29) reprinted with permission from 1985 AOTA Calendar.

Chapter 4 opening photo (p. 43) from UfaBizPhoto via Shutterstock.

Chapter 5 opening photo (p. 57) from photofort 77 via Shutterstock.

Chapter 6 opening photo (p. 63) and Chapter 7 opening photo (p. 71) reprinted with permission from 1988 AOTA Calendar.

Chapter 8 opening photo (p. 75) reprinted with permission from 1987 AOTA Calendar.

Chapter 9 opening photo (p. 81) from ABO PHOTOGRAPHY via Shutterstock.

Chapter 10 opening photo (p. 85) reprinted with permission from 1984 AOTA Calendar.

Chapter 11 opening photo (p. 89) from SpeedKingz via Shutterstock.

ACKNOWLEDGMENTS

We acknowledge our mentors, colleagues, and students in occupational therapy who have shaped our philosophy and thoughts regarding clinical practice.

ABOUT THE AUTHORS

Franklin Stein, PhD, OTR/L, FAOTA, is professor emeritus of occupational therapy at the University of South Dakota, founding editor of *Annals of International Occupational Therapy,* and life member of the American Psychological Association. He earned his Bachelor of Science in psychology from Brooklyn College, and his certificate and master's degree in occupational therapy and his PhD in counseling psychology from New York University.

Early in his career, he worked as a social worker for the New York City Department of Welfare, an occupational therapist in the New York State Psychiatric Institute, and the director of occupational therapy at the Brooklyn Day Hospital. He has been a consultant to the Hayden Residential School for Disadvantaged Youth in Boston, United Cerebral Palsy in Massachusetts, the Walter E. Fernald Developmental Center in Boston, as well as a part-time occupational therapist at Bird S. Coler Rehabilitation Hospital in New York City. He also worked as a counseling psychologist at Queens College in New York City. Previously, he was the director of the School of Medical Rehabilitation at the University of Manitoba in Winnipeg, Canada; director of the Occupational Therapy Program at the University of Wisconsin, Milwaukee; and associate professor, graduate division, at Sargent College, Boston University.

He is the first author with Kristine Haertl of *Pocket Guide to Interventions in Occupational Therapy, Second Edition* (2019); second author with Martin Rice and George Tomlin of *Clinical Research in Occupational Therapy, Sixth Edition* (2019); first author with Ingrid Soderback, Susan Cutler, and Barbara Larson of *Occupational Therapy and Ergonomics: Applying Ergonomic Principles to Everyday Occupation in the Home and at Work* (2006); first author with Susan Cutler of *Psychosocial Occupational Therapy: A Holistic Approach, Second Edition* (2002); first author with Becky Roose of *Pocket Guide to Treatment in Occupational Therapy* (2000); author of *Stress Management Questionnaire* (2003); and more than 50 publications in journals and books related to rehabilitation and psychosocial research. He has also presented more than 100 seminars, workshops, institutes, short courses, and research papers at national and international conferences in Australia, Brazil, Canada, Costa Rica, England, Finland, Mexico, Norway, Sweden, and Trinidad.

Franklin has been married to Jennie for more than 50 years and has three children: David, a physician; Jessie, an artist; and Barbara, an occupational therapist.

Kathlyn L. Reed, PhD, OTR, FAOTA, MLIS, is associate professor emerita, School of Occupational Therapy, Texas Woman's University, Houston Center, Texas. She completed her basic education in occupational therapy at the University of Kansas, earned her master's degree in occupational therapy from Western Michigan University, obtained a doctorate in special education from the University of Washington, and was awarded a second master's in information and library studies from the University of Oklahoma.

She has been active in occupational therapy for more than 50 years as a practitioner, educator, and consultant. She was a staff therapist in psychiatry at the University of Kansas Medical Center, instructor in occupational therapy at the University of Washington in Seattle, founding director of the occupational therapy program at the University of Oklahoma, and a reference and education librarian at the Houston Academy of Medicine–Texas Medical Center Library.

Reed has authored or co-authored seven textbooks, including as the second author with Lori Andersen of *The History of Occupational Therapy: The First Century* (2017); author of *Quick Reference to Occupational Therapy, Third Edition* (2014); second author with Julie Pauls of *Quick Reference to Physical Therapy, Second Edition* (2004); first author with Sharon Sanderson of *Concept of Occupational Therapy, Fourth Edition* (1999); second author with Sally Pore of *Quick Reference to Speech-Language Pathology* (1999); first author with Sandra Cunningham of *Internet Guide for Rehabilitation Professionals* (1997); and author of *Models of Practice in Occupational Therapy* (1984). She was a named a fellow of the American Occupational Therapy Association (AOTA) in 1975, received the AOTA Award of Merit in 1983, and presented the Eleanor Clarke Slagle lectureship at the AOTA annual conference in 1986. She has served in the AOTA Delegate and Representative Assemblies representing the state associations of Washington, Oklahoma, and Texas, and was chair of the AOTA Ethics Commission.

In addition, Reed is a member of the Texas Occupational Therapy Association, the World Federation of Occupational Therapists, and the Society for the Study of Occupation. She has presented at international, national, state, and local conferences, and has conducted workshops. Her interests include tracking assessments developed by occupational therapists, analyzing models of practice in occupational therapy, and studying the philosophy and history of the profession.

PREFACE

I have been an occupational therapist for a lifelong career. Occupational therapy has not only provided me with a profession, but it has also given me a philosophy to live by.

I first learned about occupational therapy when I was 21 years old, and I had just graduated from Brooklyn College. Coming from a working-class family, it seemed inevitable that I would work in a social service occupation either for the federal, state, or city government. This was the accustomed route for a student graduating from a city university. Shortly after graduating from college, when idealism met reality, I had my first encounter with occupational therapy.

I visited a state hospital for patients with mental disorders to explore the possibility of working temporarily as an aide and going to graduate school at night. The outside of the hospital had metal bars on the window balconies. Inside, I saw distressing individuals in worn-out clothing, some of them frantically pacing, others gesturing, expressing themselves in a way I found difficult to understand. When I toured the occupational therapy department, I observed that the occupational therapists used arts and crafts in a shop-like atmosphere. The patients were actively engaged and seemed to enjoy what they were doing. I was very impressed by the commitment of the occupational therapists working with the patients, and I could perceive myself doing exactly what the occupational therapists were carrying out. I saw that occupational therapy was a humane way to work with people who had a severe mental illness. The visit left an enormous impression on me. I became highly motivated to become an occupational therapist, and I started on my graduate education at night at New York University while working full-time as a social worker for the New York City Department of Welfare.

As I learned about occupational therapy, it demonstrated to me that it is a profession based on helping individuals cope with their disabilities by using purposeful and meaningful activities as interventions. The philosophy of occupational therapy is based on a humanistic approach where we view each individual as being unique and having innate abilities that can be positively developed. We perceive that people have intrinsic capacities that can be fostered so as to improve their lives and reach their potential, and so that an individual with a mental illness can become engaged in a gratifying and enjoyable activity, such as learning how to paint, composing poetry, working in ceramics, or learning photography. This same approach can be applied to oneself as a way to bring about one's maximum potential. My parents came from immigrant families, and I was the first person in my family to obtain a college degree. I was fortunate enough to have opportunities that I took advantage of. I believe in this philosophy, and I have applied it to my own life in my education by obtaining a master's degree in occupational therapy and a PhD in psychology. I have applied this philosophy in becoming a clinician, professor, author, consultant, and researcher in occupational therapy.

—*Franklin Stein, PhD, OTR/L, FAOTA*

My career in occupational therapy began when my father overheard two occupational therapists talking shop while eating at a restaurant in Grand Rapids, Michigan. In his mind, their discussion of the crafts and games they were using with the children referred to occupational therapy seemed to fit my abilities and interests. I was 13. Although many other careers were brought to my attention during my high school years in Rockford, Illinois, none seemed to fit any better. My hands worked better than my brain, so I needed a profession that applied knowledge and skills rather than one that advanced great ideas. My father was a research chemist and inventor. Following in his footsteps did not seem feasible. My mother was an English literature major, and I did not like Shakespeare. She did know how to do needlework and weaving activities, and how to play card and table games, which she willingly taught me.

As my senior year in high school approached, two choices of occupational therapy programs were identified as close by: one in Chicago, Illinois, and the other in Madison, Wisconsin. Since my parents were now living in Beloit, Wisconsin, I could qualify to pay in-state tuition, so my choice was to attend the University of Wisconsin. After 3 years in Madison, I transferred to the University of Kansas in Lawrence to become a Jayhawker (a mythical bird mascot), to join my mother's sorority, and to graduate from the same school my parents had attended—birds of a feather.

My first job was as a staff psychiatric occupational therapist in Kansas City, Kansas, at the University of Kansas Medical Center. At the state occupational therapy association meetings, there was discussion about occupational therapists moving to master's level entry, and I did not want to be left behind, so I applied to the master's program at Western Michigan University in Kalamazoo. My timing was a bit off. My master's degree was awarded 33 years ahead of the 1999 resolution adopted by the American Occupational Therapy Association that would require master's level entry for all occupational therapists.

While at Western Michigan, the faculty encouraged me to consider teaching. Upon graduation, I applied for a position on the faculty at the University of Washington in Seattle. Faculty positions often require a doctorate, so I enrolled in the doctoral program in special education because, at that time, there was no doctoral program in occupational therapy. Upon graduation, I accepted a position with the University of Oklahoma Health Sciences Center in Oklahoma City to start a school of occupational therapy. When the new school started, Oklahoma was home to about 40 occupational therapists, of which about 20 were employed. My time was split between teaching students and consulting with hospitals, clinics, and nursing homes to develop or update occupational therapy service programs. A major issue was to convince administrators that occupational therapists did more than make ceramic objects by pouring slip clay into plaster models and glazing the clay items the models produced. Another issue was to improve the quality of the textbooks the students were reading. So, while at the University of Oklahoma, I co-authored my first textbook on occupational therapy and also became interested in understanding the history of occupational therapy.

To locate early articles on occupational therapy, I had to learn to be a better library user. I enrolled in the librarian program and received a second master's degree in library and information studies. With my library degree in hand, I took a breather from occupational therapy and became a reference and education librarian at the Houston Academy of Medicine–Texas Medical Center library in Houston, Texas. The occupational therapy program at the Texas Woman's University campus in Houston was directly across the street from the library, and the faculty quickly convinced me to teach a course at Texas Woman's University. After several years of dividing my time between being a librarian and an occupational therapy instructor, I returned to teaching occupational therapy full-time. Since retirement from faculty life, most of my time has been occupied in authoring or co-authoring articles and textbooks and in continuing to present at local, state, national, and international meetings.

In writing this guide to occupational therapy, as authors who have had satisfying lifetime careers as occupational therapists, we want to share our enthusiasm for the profession and to help guide those who are considering occupational therapy as a career.

—*Kathlyn L. Reed, PhD, OTR, FAOTA, MLIS*

FOREWORD

Years ago, as a high school student entering my final year at an American school in Germany, I had the good fortune to hear the words "occupational therapist" for the very first time. Oddly enough, this introduction did not occur through a book, a guidance counselor, or a chance meeting. Instead, it arrived through a character in a movie (Rossen, 1964) that was portraying an occupational therapist working in a psychiatric hospital. This was during the time when many such facilities existed, with most now having long been bulldozed (both physically and metaphorically) in the name of "progress."

It turns out that, quite by coincidence, I was then especially attentive to career opportunities, having been assigned a term paper by a wise teacher of philosophy and literature. She had directed the class to reflect on how we might match our personal values with our career aspirations. But, I had not yet settled on a career choice. For some reason, perhaps borne of adolescent rebellion or independence, I had resisted the urgings of my mother to pursue a career in medicine. I was more interested in the humanities, and in psychology and sociology.

The result of this chance exposure to a new possibility motivated me to contact the American Occupational Therapy Association (AOTA) for career information. Some weeks later (this was during the pre-Internet era), I received a letter with a small brochure with some brief information and a list of 30 or so universities in the United States with accredited programs (there are hundreds now). The rest of the story is history, having played out over a half century in an engaging and rewarding association with this "emerging" profession that is now over a century old. My decision to pursue occupational therapy studies would have been far better informed had a useful guide like this book been available at that time.

There has been much change in the profession during my career, most of it (but not all) for the better. For example, men constitute a larger number of the profession's members than they did then—a good thing if one believes (as do I) that the demographics of a field should mirror those of the clients it serves. Unfortunately, while the gender distribution is modestly improved in the United States, ethnic diversity remains a significant challenge (AOTA, 2019). Another change is in the profession's startling recent growth. The sheer number of professionals in the field nationally and globally has mushroomed over the past 3 decades, driven both by the growth in health care generally but also by a growing awareness of the benefits of employing occupational therapists in a very wide range of traditional and less common settings.

A third major change involves the scientific advancement of the field's body of knowledge. Motivated by plans from within the profession as well as by the public expectation that health care should now be evidenced-based, occupational therapy has encouraged the development of a strong network of clinical scientists who have worked to evolve the field's theory and practice through systematic research (Christiansen, 1983). While much work remains to be done, the purposeful development of this robust research community has arguably and notably increased the field's standing as a "science-driven, evidence-based" practice profession (AOTA, 2007). The foresight of occupational therapy leaders a half-century ago to create a charitable and scientific foundation to support such research efforts can be seen now as remarkably wise.

This scientific progress has been supported by changes in educational programs, often following hotly debated decisions within the profession to require that entry-level therapists earn graduate degrees. Most recently, the debate has centered on a requirement for new therapists to earn a doctoral degree. However, the field has most recently (and reasonably, I think) taken the position that its health care delivery aims can be accomplished with multiple routes of entry at the post-baccalaureate level. Perhaps ultimately, all professional-level educational programs in the field will evolve toward doctoral education as a natural progression. But this will depend on a host of factors not entirely decided by the profession itself.

That said, one might argue that a more important question is, "What can the field's graduates provide that adds value to efforts that address the social and health needs of society?" Here, perhaps, is where prospective students or employers of occupational therapy personnel may wish to take notice because I contend that this added value is both unique and important.

Occupational therapy emerged from social movements with moral and humanitarian roots (Bing, 1981). Its leading advocates in the United States came from callings as diverse as nursing, medicine, psychiatry, social work, architecture, and vocational rehabilitation (Andersen & Reed, 2017). At its core, the notion was that the daily occupations, or purposeful and meaningful activities of humans, not only reflect the state of their health but also contribute to it. In ideal occupational therapy, each therapeutic encounter is thus tailored in the context of a particular client's life situation, aimed at focusing on the tasks and underlying abilities that are ultimately important and meaningful to the client. Many argue that authentic occupational therapy pays close attention to this detail, recognizing that knowing the client's story leads to therapy that is relevant and thus helps build a "bridge of understanding" between the personal world of the client and the unfamiliar realms of social or biological medicine (Engelhardt, 1983).

Unfortunately, the efficiency demands of profit-driven health care have sometimes resulted in the use of "one size fits all" protocols for therapy. One result is the emergence of the term "occupation-based intervention." This category itself is disturbing evidence of a deviation from the personalized therapy of the past because it suggests that some interventions are not occupation-based. Indeed, the field's founding name was proudly derived from having occupation as its signature style of "curing" (Yerxa, 1998). If the profession strays too far from its founding ideals, it could diminish the effectiveness and uniqueness of its services and erode its full value to society (Shannon, 1977). This is not just nostalgic rhetoric; it is borne out by controlled clinical research (Gutman et al., 2019).

In the coming years, there will continue to be great changes in occupational therapy as practiced in the United States. Some of these will be necessitated by the health care infrastructure, which will be forced to change by the unsustainable economic burden of a costly and inefficient profit-driven system (Chassin & Galvin, 1998). As this is being written, the world is being challenged and changed at warp speed by the coronavirus (COVID-19) pandemic, perhaps destined to be one of the major global events in history. In the United States, the pandemic has revealed systematic weaknesses in the nation's social, health care, and economic infrastructures. These weaknesses and their consequences will undoubtedly lead to requests for significant changes in societal structures once the pandemic is over.

Even before this crisis, one could have easily foreseen dramatic changes in society resulting from rapid developments in science and technology. Genetic medicine remains in its infancy, and digital technologies are changing the way health care is delivered. These advances will most assuredly affect the roles of some occupational therapists, yet create opportunities for others, particularly when it comes to humanizing care that too often seems corporate, sterile, and impersonal. Change brings opportunity, and there will always be a market for the brand of quality care that results when clients feel involved and respected as individuals rather than as faceless insurance cardholders.

No one knows with certainty what changes will occur in the years ahead. But whatever evolves, it seems certain that with wise leadership (and an appreciation for history), the profession can maintain its flexibility and adapt to change. With creative imagination, and recognition of the unmeasurable value of enabling people to engage in the roles, tasks, and activities that bring meaning to their lives, the field will remain on solid footing. After all, "people are healthy or diseased in terms of the activities open to them or denied them", according to insightful medical philosopher Tristram Engelhardt, Jr. (1977).

As you read this useful guide, authored by respected authorities with unparalleled experience and wisdom, I trust that these beginning thoughts from a veteran inside observer will assist you in better understanding and appreciating the larger context of the profession. Occupational therapy has a storied and distinguished past, and I have always maintained that its best years lie beyond the horizons we are fast approaching.

—*Charles Christiansen, EdD, OTR, FAOTA*

Dr. Christiansen is a clinical professor of occupational therapy at The University of Texas Medical Branch at Galveston. He currently serves as Chair, Board of Directors, Society for the Study of Occupation:USA. During his full-time professional career, he served as CEO of the American Occupational Therapy Foundation from 2007 until 2015. Prior to that, he held administrative leadership roles at the University of Minnesota, The University of Texas Medical Branch, the University of British Columbia, and other institutions. He received the Award of Merit, its highest honor, from the American Occupational Therapy Association in 2017, during its centennial year. He lives with his wife, Beth Jones, PhD, in Rochester, Minnesota, where they operate Bella Vista Farm, a boarding and training facility for dressage horses and their owners.

REFERENCES

American Occupational Therapy Association. (2007). AOTA's Centennial Vision and executive summary. *American Journal of Occupational Therapy, 61*(6), 613-614. https://doi.org/10.5014/ajot.61.6.613

American Occupational Therapy Association (February, 2019). Unpublished report. Special Task Force on External Issues. American Occupational Therapy Association. https://www.aota.org/~/media/Corporate/Files/AboutAOTA/BOD/Special-Task-Force-February-2019-Summary-Report.pdf

Andersen, L. T., & Reed, K. L. (2017). *The history of occupational therapy: The first century.* Thorofare, NJ: SLACK Incorporated.

Bing, R. K. (1981). Occupational therapy: A paraphrastic journey. *American Journal of Occupational Therapy, 35*(8), 499-518. https://doi.org/10.5014/ajot.35.8.499

Chassin, M. R., & Galvin, R. W. (1998). The urgent need to improve health care quality: Institute of Medicine National Roundtable on Health Care Quality. *Journal of the American Medical Association, 280*(11), 1000-1005. https://doi:10.1001/jama.280.11.1000

Christiansen, C. (1983). Research: An economic imperative. *Occupation, Participation and Health, 3*(4), 195-198. https://doi.org/10.1177/153944928300300401

Engelhardt, H. T. (1977). Defining occupational therapy: The meaning of therapy and the virtues of occupation. *American Journal of Occupational Therapy, 31*(10), 666-672. https://ajot.aota.org/

Engelhardt, H. T. (1983). Occupational therapists as technologists and custodians of meaning. In G. Kielhofner (Ed.), *Health through occupation: Theory and practice in occupational therapy* (pp. 139-145). Philadelphia, PA: F. A. Davis Company.

Gutman, S., Balasubramanian, S., Herzog, M., Kim, E., Swirnow, H., Retig, Y., & Wolff, S. (2019). Effectiveness of a tailored intervention for women with ADHD and ADHD symptoms: A randomized controlled study. *American Journal of Occupational Therapy, 73*(4 Suppl. 1), 7311520394p1-7311520394p1. https://doi.org/10.5014/ajot.2019.73S1-PO2035

Rossen, R (Director). (1964). *Lilith* [Film]. Columbia Pictures.

Shannon, P. (1977). The derailment of occupational therapy. *American Journal of Occupational Therapy, 26*, 229-234.

Yerxa, E. J. (1998). Occupation: The keystone of a curriculum for a self-defined profession. *American Journal of Occupational Therapy, 52*(5), 365-372. https://doi.org/10.5014/ajot.52.5.365

INTRODUCTION

Occupational therapy is one of the world's fastest-growing professions. According to the World Federation of Occupational Therapists, about 580,000 occupational therapists are practicing in more than 90 countries (https://www.wfot.org). In the United States, there are about 143,300 occupational therapists (https://www.bls.gov/ooh/healthcare/occupational-therapists.htm).

Occupational therapy as a profession was founded in 1917 in the United States during the first World War to provide curative and diversional activities for soldiers with disabilities who were making the transition from military hospitals back into the community. At that time, the therapists were called *reconstruction aides* or *Gray Ladies* because they wore gray uniforms. They were nurses, social workers, and librarians with knowledge of handicrafts and good interpersonal skills who helped the soldiers engage in craft activities, such as art, ceramics, knitting, weaving, and bead work. The activities helped motivate the soldiers to improve and helped reduce the severe stress and anxieties of war. From this beginning, occupational therapy has developed into a complex health care profession that requires graduate education and provides health care services, such as retraining in the essential everyday activities or occupations of living for people with physical, psychological, and cognitive disabilities.

In this book, we will explain what occupational therapy is, describe the history of occupational therapy, discuss the specific interventions that occupational therapists use in their daily work, detail the educational requirements for becoming an occupational therapist, highlight the clinical settings where occupational therapists work, and explain the types of positions and specialty areas that occupational therapists engage in and the future prospects.

Purpose

The major aims of this book are:

- To describe the profession of occupational therapy to students interested in a health care profession, health consumers, and caregivers and family members, so they can understand what occupational therapists do in helping people function in their everyday activities.
- To educate prospective students in high school or college about occupational therapy so they can learn more about occupational therapy, the personal qualities needed to be an effective occupational therapy

clinician, educational requirements in becoming an occupational therapist, and the prospects for employment.

- To assist high school and college counselors to provide up-to-date information to students who might be interested in pursuing a career in occupational therapy.
- To provide detailed information on how occupational therapists perform their jobs, such as in hospitals, clinics, or schools; the occupational therapy scope of practice; and research supporting interventions for advocates of occupational therapy.
- To provide a glossary of terms that would help students, consumers, and advocates understand the profession.

Questions to Guide the Writing of This Book

- What is the education of occupational therapists?
- How do they differ from physical therapists and other health professionals?
- How do they plan treatments?
- How do they evaluate the effectiveness of treatment?
- How are occupational therapists referred for treatment?
- Does a doctor have to prescribe occupational therapy?
- What skills do you need to become an occupational therapist?
- Are there treatment protocols like in medicine?
- What are the personal skills of an occupational therapist?
- Are occupational therapy services covered by Medicare? Medicaid? Private insurance?
- What do occupational therapists do in public schools?
- How do occupational therapists differ from special education teachers?
- Why do occupational therapists use splinting?
- What do occupational therapists know about holistic medicine?
- What is a typical day like for an occupational therapist working in acute rehabilitation in a hospital?
- What type of documentation do occupational therapists do when assessing patient progress and testing for activities of daily life skills?
- Do occupational therapists work with people with mental disorders?
- What is the difference between registered occupational therapists and certified occupational therapy assistants?
- How did occupational therapy begin as a health profession?

- Do occupational therapists work in the Army, Navy, Air Force, and Coast Guard?
- Can occupational therapists work overseas?
- What are the specialty areas of occupational therapy?
- Who are the people with disabilities that occupational therapists assist?
- What is a typical workday for an occupational therapist working in a hospital?
- What are the opportunities in clinical practice, teaching, administration, and research?
- What are the average salaries for occupational therapists?
- What are the future trends in occupational therapy?
- What are the definitions of terms regarding occupational therapy?
- What are the personal characteristics of occupational therapists?
- Where can you learn about occupational therapy?
- How do you become an occupational therapist?
- What are the typical courses that an occupational therapist takes in college?
- How do you become a certified occupational therapy assistant?
- Which United States universities offer programs in occupational therapy?
- What are the average costs for obtaining a degree in occupational therapy?

A Philosophy of Occupational Therapy

- The diversity of individuals regarding gender, race, religion, ethnic origins, and sexual orientation must be respected.
- Every individual has the right to obtain the best health care available.
- The disability should not identify the individual; the unique person does (people-first language).
- The environment should be adjusted to help the individual with a disability become maximally functional.
- The potential abilities of an individual should be encouraged through support and opportunities to engage in purposeful and meaningful activities.
- Every individual, no matter how severely disabled, has the right to be treated with dignity.

- Children with disabilities should have the right to be educated in integrated classrooms.

- People with disabilities have the right to work and to use their abilities to the maximum.

- Universal design should be encouraged in public places to reduce barriers and allow, for example, individuals in wheelchairs access to buildings.

- Prevention of disabilities and diseases through encouraging smoking cessation, exercise, good nutrition, and stress management should be a prime aim of government interventions.

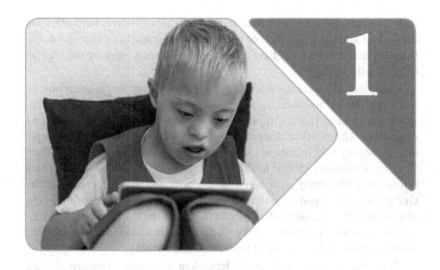

What Is Occupational Therapy?

Occupational therapy is a health profession to help people of all ages with disabilities to function in their everyday occupations by using activities and interventions for therapeutic purposes. Occupational therapy is also a dynamic and evolving profession. The scope of practice is always widening where occupational therapists, for example, engage in interventions to prevent diseases and occupational injuries. To be successful as an occupational therapist, one has to have knowledge in the basic and social sciences—such as anatomy, physiology, kinesiology, and psychology—to be familiar with the medical sciences and understand the dynamics of disabilities, such as stroke, spinal cord injury, cerebral palsy, and schizophrenia.

In addition, the occupational therapist has to learn the interventions that are applied in treatment and analyze the steps in reteaching an everyday skill to a person with a disability. The occupational therapist has to have the interpersonal skills to develop rapport and to motivate patients to use all

Stein, F., & Reed, K. L.
Occupational Therapy: A Guide for Prospective Students, Consumers, and Advocates (pp. 1-5).
© 2021 Taylor & Francis Group.

their capabilities for improvement to occur. Rehabilitation is hard work for the patient and the therapist. For occupational therapy to be successful, the therapist and patient must have a therapeutic alliance, working together to help the patient improve.

Occupational therapists work as teachers in helping people learn how to live a healthy life and assisting in making the home environment or workspace safe, and as healers in helping people cope with their illnesses and disabilities. They work in diverse settings, such as neonatal clinics in hospitals where they help infants who are premature develop sensory skills. They work in community mental health centers to help individuals with mental illness cope effectively with everyday stressors and develop coping skills. Occupational therapists also work in nursing homes and independent living situations to help people with dementia use as much of their cognitive function as possible. Additionally, they work in public schools to help students adapt best to the classroom and to enable their learning.

Occupational therapy is an independent profession concerned with health and well-being that cooperates with physicians, nurses, psychologists, educators, physical therapists, speech language pathologists, and others to promote healthy living, improve quality of life, and reduce the impact of disability. Occupational therapists often provide rehabilitation services in conjunction with physical therapists and speech language pathologists to help people with disabilities gain or regain everyday functions, such as the ability to dress, bathe, feed themselves, communicate effectively, and ambulate and move their muscles. Occupational therapists also work with psychologists, social workers, and special education teachers to help people with developmental disabilities cope effectively with activities of daily living and participate in school and educational activities. In addition, occupational therapists may provide consultation and education to employers and community planners to improve the safety and efficiency of work settings and communities to reduce the potential for injury and loss of ability to participate in everyday life.

There are two levels of entry into the profession. The registered occupational therapist (OTR) now requires a master's degree to practice, whereas a certified occupational therapy assistant (COTA) requires an associate degree, which is equivalent to 2 years of college, such as in a community college. Both the occupational therapist and the occupational therapy assistant are required to pass a national administered examination to practice. After passing the national examination, they are able to use the title OTR or COTA. In addition, to practice in a specific state, the OTR and COTA need to pass a licensing examination administered by a state licensing board.

How will you know that occupational therapy is the right choice of profession for you? Choosing a career after high school or while in college is a significant decision. Each of the authors of this book has spent a lifetime as an occupational therapist. We have had positions as occupational therapy clinicians working directly with patients in hospitals and clinics. We have been teachers and professors in universities, consultants to occupational therapy programs, administrators of occupational therapy departments, and clinical researchers. We have presented papers at national and international conferences and have visited occupational therapy departments throughout the world.

Occupational therapy is a correct career choice if you enjoy working directly with people, have a curiosity about health and medicine, want to help people with disabilities reach their maximum potential, and are willing to be a lifelong learner. Occupational therapy is a social service profession, like medicine, nursing, psychology, social work, physical therapy, and speech language pathology and audiology. It is a humanistic profession in that we are concerned about the whole person and how the person develops as a mature human being with unique interests and abilities.

Occupational therapy is similar to other helping professions. In deciding upon occupational therapy as a career, you must consider whether you can picture yourself carrying through the tasks that occupational therapists do every day in their encounters with patients. Occupational therapy is also a dynamic field, in that occupational therapists work in diverse settings, such as public schools, hospitals, community clinics, and, recently, in private practice. The profession offers many opportunities for advancement, such as becoming an administrator, director of a clinical program, university professor, clinical researcher, or academic fieldwork supervisor. There are also expanding opportunities for positions in foreign countries as occupational therapists and university instructors.

As occupational therapists, we focus on a person's ability to perform the everyday tasks of living, the leisure activities of an individual, and the factors at work that bring job satisfaction. Occupational therapy is also an evolving profession in terms of the scope of practice and education. The profession has changed dramatically in the last 100 years. The entry-level education in the United States has progressed from a technical degree in the 1920s to a bachelor's degree, to now a master's degree requirement, and, in the near future, to an entry-level doctorate in occupational therapy. In addition to the expanding roles of occupational therapy, the scope of practice has also widened to include work in neonatal units, cognitive therapy for people with dementia, and forensic occupational therapy in penal institutions. In the pages that follow, we discuss in detail the many components of occupational therapy that make up the profession, from history to the current scope of practice.

The following is a description of an occupational therapist's daily routine.

A DAY IN THE LIFE OF AN ACUTE CARE OCCUPATIONAL THERAPIST IN A LARGE URBAN HOSPITAL

I work in a large 400-bed hospital in a suburb of Los Angeles. As I arrive at work, I'm greeted by my fellow therapists, and I take a seat at my desk in a multi-office room. I make note of any special meetings for the day and put on my lab coat. The schedule is placed on a large board with paper copies for each therapist. All the patients on occupational therapy service are listed and assigned a therapist for the day. Assignments are usually made by the therapy manager. I take my list and sit by an open computer. I first log on and check my work email. News of upcoming meetings, surveys, and student assignments is communicated here. Next, I create my list of patients and begin my chart reviews. A typical day consists of six evaluations and one treatment, or four evaluations and five treatments. Usually, these are all new clients, so a thorough chart review is essential.

After about 30 minutes, it's time to head up to the floors and begin seeing patients. I also carry a hospital cellphone to allow my boss to contact me with any changes in schedule. Therapists work closely with the nurses to coordinate appropriate treatment times and exchange information regarding the patient's status. The occupational therapist may be working on several different floors and needs to be efficient with their time. On a typical day you may see patients in critical care, pediatrics, the intensive care unit, the cardiac unit, or the orthopedic unit. The hospital also has an outpatient department and an acute rehab unit, which pull therapists from inpatient acute care when needed. Diagnoses range among stroke, brain injury, heart attack, respiratory failure, joint replacements, and multi-trauma. Patients may be on ventilators or have heart monitors, intravenous therapies, drains, catheters, or wound vacuum-assisted closures. Some patients are newly hemiplegic, paraplegic, or brain-injured. Presentation may be confused, lethargic, depressed, disoriented, agitated, or in pain.

The therapist introduces themself to the client and educates them on the purpose and importance of occupational therapy. Depending on the patient's ability to respond, a history of prior level of function, career, hobbies, and current living status is obtained. Next, the patient is asked to describe how they are feeling, any pain, nausea, or dizziness. Vital signs are taken to ensure the patient is safe to move. Next, the patient is assisted to sit at the edge of the bed, with the therapist making note of bed mobility and sitting balance. The occupational therapist then assesses vision, upper extremity range of motion, coordination, and strength. If safe to do so, the next step may be to transfer the patient to a bedside commode or ambulate with a walker to the bathroom. Grooming tasks are also assessed either standing at the sink or sitting at the edge of the bed with a tray table in front of the patient. Throughout the mobility phase, the therapist is mindful of any tubes or wires attached to the patient. Safety awareness is the primary concern. Once returning to the bed or chair, the therapist may assess dressing skills with slipper socks and a hospital gown. If appropriate, family may be asked to bring in comfortable clothing for the patient to practice dressing in the next session. The occupational therapist also builds rapport by expressing care through healing touch, active listening, and encouraging and reassuring the patient throughout the whole therapy session.

At the end of the session, the patient is left in a safe position with the call light and all essentials within reach. The patient's performance is communicated to the nurse, physical therapist, and speech therapist if available. Documentation is done on the computer, and the evaluation is completed and sent to the ordering physician. After all the patients are seen for the day, the occupational therapist completes any unfinished documentation and clocks out for the day.

—*Barbara Plato, BS, OTR/L*
Occupational Therapist
Northridge Hospital
Los Angeles, California

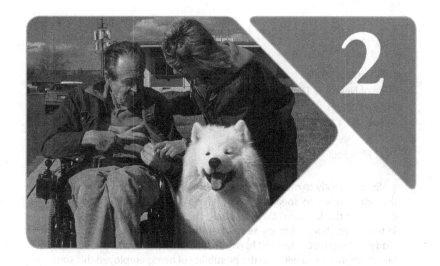

Learning About
Occupational Therapy

When I (FS) graduated from Brooklyn College with a major in psychology, I spoke to a college counselor regarding available positions. I was interested in a social service career, such as social work or psychology. He referred me to a job opening as an occupational therapy instructor at Brooklyn State Hospital. I had no idea what an occupational therapy instructor did. This was 1956, and about 5,000 occupational therapists were employed in the United States, with perhaps a dozen countries that had occupational therapists (http://stats.bisgov/oco/). In contrast, in 2019 there were more than 140,000 occupational therapists in the United States (https://www.bls.gov/ooh/healthcare/occupational-therapists.htm) and about 580,000 occupational therapists in more than 90 countries (https://www.wfot.org).

Following is a verbatim account of a letter that I sent in 1958 to the director of occupational therapy at New York State Department of Mental Hygiene, where I was applying for a full New York University scholarship, which I subsequently received.

Stein, F., & Reed, K. L.
*Occupational Therapy: A Guide for Prospective
Students, Consumers, and Advocates* (pp. 7-28).
© 2021 Taylor & Francis Group.

4/28/1958

Miss Virginia Scullin
State of New York Department of Mental Hygiene
217 Lark Street
Albany, NY 12229

Dear Miss Scullin,

Subsequently to meeting you at Columbia University on April 8, I had the opportunity to speak to Mr. William Roash (occupational therapy director at the Brooklyn Day Hospital). The prevocational arrangement in the occupational therapy section of the hospital, I learned, is a pilot study and the first of its kind in psychiatric rehabilitation in this country. Mr. Roash discussed with me the possibility of being employed this summer as a trainee. I explained to Mr. Roash my interest in psychiatric occupational therapy and my desire to work in this area following my course of study at New York University. I completed a form for a scholarship stipend and forwarded it to Mr. Roash. I called the hospital today, and I have learned that Mr. Roash is out on sick leave. I do not know, therefore, if my application has been forwarded to you.

I became acquainted with the field of occupational therapy after graduating from Brooklyn College in January 1956, at which time I received a Bachelor of Science degree in psychology. I visited the occupational therapy shops at Brooklyn State Hospital and noticed the relationship between the craft media and therapy. The therapist with a knowledge of psychiatry and crafts is an essential person in the rehabilitation program. The possibilities and potential of occupational therapy seemed great. During the spring of 1956, I entered New York University as a part-time certificate student. I am currently enrolled full-time carrying 18 credits this semester. I will need 20 credits to complete my course requirements.

Occupational therapy is important to me since it would allow me to integrate my interests in music, drama, and art with my background in psychology. The use of music therapy in psychiatric hospitals will give me the opportunity to develop what I believe has great potential. The possibility of presenting "unstructured" dramas and musicals in a hospital can be included in a rehabilitation program. The dynamics and therapeutic aid of painting and watercolor can also play an important role in occupational therapy. Through the broadening of creative interests, an individual's capacities can be realized. In the mental hospital, the therapist can help the patient to explore his own abilities and aid him in expression. The therapist is part of a team in a psychiatric hospital composed of a psychiatrist, psychologist, social worker, nurse, and attendant, which gives him the experience to exchange ideas regarding treatment and care of the patient. The therapist can also create warm relationships with the patient, which brings gratification to both.

My experience in life during the last 10 years has been enriched with friends and jobs. During my high school and college years, I had worked part-time and summers as a salesman, postal clerk, waiter, office boy, play street director for the Police Athletic League, and children's counselor. These jobs have given me financial independence and a sense of responsibility. My parents have been very important in encouraging me to assess my plans. From May 1956 until January 1958, I was employed as a social worker for the New York City Department of Welfare. This experience has aided me in my relationships with other people in a useful service. Although I am 24, I think that my employment experiences and education have given me a mature outlook.

I look with zeal and great interest in being considered for a scholarship stipend and employment by the Department of Mental Hygiene. Thank you for your kind consideration in this matter.

Very truly yours,
Franklin Stein

As I look back on this letter that was written more than 60 years ago, I see myself as an ambitious young man eager to begin a social service profession. What comes across is the honesty and drive to become an occupational therapist. I was living with my parents in a three-room apartment in Brooklyn, New York. My parents came from immigrant families from Romania, and my father had an unskilled job as a gas station attendant earning a meager salary. Finishing college and becoming an occupational therapist was the American Dream come true. I completed my academic requirements in 1959 after clinical internships at the Bronx Veterans Administration Hospital, where I gained experience with patients with spinal cord injuries and general, medical, and surgical conditions. I also did internships in psychiatry at Buffalo State Hospital, Buffalo Children's Hospital, and the San Fernando Veterans Administration tuberculosis hospital in California.

After receiving my certificate in occupational therapy, I passed the National Board for Certification in Occupational Therapy (NBCOT) exam, which entitled me to use the title registered occupational therapist

(OTR). My first position was as an occupational therapist at New York State Psychiatric Institute. After working as a clinician and consultant in occupational therapy for 8 years, I became a professor at Boston University. I have had a full career with sabbaticals in Cambridge University in England, the University of Alberta and McGill University in Canada, and Uppsala University in Sweden. I have also presented lectures throughout the world.

What can be derived now from my early experience in learning about occupational therapy? First, the field of occupational therapy has changed dramatically in the last 60 years. In the late 1950s, occupational therapists worked in general hospitals, curative and sheltered workshops, home service, mental hospitals, tuberculosis hospitals and sanitaria, children's hospitals and schools for children with disabilities, Army and Navy hospitals, and hospitals of the Veterans Administration (McNary, 1954). Craft activities, such as art, ceramics, weaving, basketry, woodwork, and jewelry-making, were used as therapeutic media. Presently, relatively few occupational therapists work in psychiatric rehabilitation facilities. According to the American Occupational Therapy Association (AOTA), most occupational therapists now work in long-term care and skilled nursing facilities, outpatient clinics, hospitals, and public and private schools. The interventions that occupational therapists employ now are numerous and tailored to the individual needs of the patient. Interventions are also assessed for efficacy through clinical research. They include, for example:

- Splinting in hand therapy for individuals recovering from hand surgery
- Sensory integration for autistic children
- Constraint therapy and mirror therapy for individuals recovering from a stroke
- Work conditioning for people who have suffered an injury at work
- Training in activities of daily living for people with disabilities
- Assistive devices for people with arthritis
- Ergonomic adaptations in the bathroom to prevent falls in the home
- Biofeedback techniques for people in a stroke rehabilitation program
- Physical agent modalities, such as ultrasounds, for pain management
- Orthosis design, fabrication, fitting, and prosthesis training for people with amputations
- Creative activities, such as art, music, poetry, dance, and crafts, with people who are experiencing mental health issues
- Cognitive stimulation programs for individuals diagnosed with Alzheimer's disease

As occupational therapy has evolved, the fields of recreational therapy, music therapy, dance therapy, and art therapy are now standard professions based on the original concepts of occupational therapy in applying creative media to help clients with disabilities and emotional problems. Some occupational therapists still use these media in their interventions. In addition, there are occupational therapists who use other interventions—such as tai chi, yoga, massage, and Rolfing—that they have acquired through certification or competency in combining these interventions with occupational therapy.

How would a high school student or college undergraduate learn about occupational therapy? Using my own example, I first went to a college counselor to discuss the career possibilities based on my academic record, personal characteristics, and interests. I also visited an occupational therapy department in a hospital to observe what occupational therapists do. Now in the computer age, much information about occupational therapy is available online.

The **AOTA** website (https://www.aota.org/) contains much information on what occupational therapy is, where occupational therapists work, and the educational requirements for becoming an occupational therapist. AOTA provides a list of colleges and universities that have approved educational programs for occupational therapists and occupational therapy assistants.

AOTA defines occupational therapy as follows.

The practice of occupational therapy means the therapeutic use of occupations, including everyday life activities with individuals, groups, populations, or organizations to support participation, performance, and function in roles and situations in home, school, workplace, community, and other settings. Occupational therapy services are provided for habilitation, rehabilitation, and the promotion of health and wellness to those who have or are at risk for developing an illness, injury, disease, disorder, condition, impairment, disability, activity limitation, or participation restriction. Occupational therapy addresses the physical, cognitive, psychosocial, sensory-perceptual, and other aspects of performance in a variety of contexts and environments to support engagement in occupations that affect physical and mental health, well-being, and quality of life.

The **World Federation of Occupational Therapists** website (https://www.wfot.org) contains valuable information on approved occupational therapy educational programs throughout the world. It defines occupational therapy within an international framework as follows.

Occupational therapy is a client-centred health profession concerned with promoting health and well-being through occupation. The primary goal of occupational therapy is to enable people to participate in the activities of everyday life. Occupational therapists achieve this outcome by working with people and communities to enhance their ability to engage in the occupations they want to, need to, or are expected to do, or by modifying the occupation or the environment to better support their occupational engagement.

Volunteering in a health facility is another way to learn about occupational therapy in high school. Hospital volunteers, for example, transport patients in wheelchairs, greet visitors to a hospital, help in clerical work, and assist nurses and aides in making patients comfortable. The volunteer may be able to observe occupational therapy interventions and perhaps assist the therapist in routine tasks.

State occupational therapy associations exist in every state in the United States. Each occupational therapy association has a licensing procedure, advocates for occupational therapy, and provides information on occupational therapy for the consumer. For example, the Wisconsin Occupational Therapy Association focuses on promotion of the profession and professional services of occupational therapists and occupational therapy assistants, as well as the education of occupational therapy students, in the state of Wisconsin.

The *Occupational Outlook Handbook* contains up-to-date occupational therapist information (Table 2-1).

TABLE 2-1. QUICK FACTS: OCCUPATIONAL THERAPISTS

Median Pay, 2019	$84,950 per year $40.84 per hour
Typical Entry-Level Education	Master's degree
Work Experience in a Related Occupation	None
On-the-Job Training	None
Number of Jobs, 2019	143,300
Job Outlook, 2019-2029	16% (Much faster than average)
Employment Change, 2019-2029	22,700
Reprinted from https://www.bls.gov/ooh/	

WHAT DO OCCUPATIONAL THERAPISTS DO?

Occupational therapists treat injured, ill, or disabled patients through the therapeutic use of everyday activities. They help these patients develop, recover, improve, and maintain the skills needed for daily living and working.

Occupational therapists typically handle the following duties:

- Review patients' medical history, ask them questions, and observe them doing tasks
- Evaluate patients' conditions and needs
- Develop treatment plans for patients, identifying specific goals and the types of activities that will be used to help the patients work toward those goals
- Help people with disabilities perform tasks, such as teaching a person who has had a stroke how to get dressed
- Demonstrate exercises—for example, stretching the joints for arthritis relief—that can help relieve pain in people with chronic conditions
- Evaluate patients' homes or workplaces and, on the basis of each patient's health needs, identify potential improvements, such as labeling kitchen cabinets for an older person with poor memory
- Educate each patient's family and employer about how to accommodate and care for the patient
- Recommend special equipment, such as wheelchairs and eating aids, and instruct patients on how to use that equipment
- Assess and record patients' activities and progress for patient evaluations, for billing, and for reporting to physicians and other health care providers
- Use telehealth to communicate with clients online

Patients with permanent disabilities, such as cerebral palsy, often need help performing daily tasks. Therapists show patients how to use appropriate adaptive equipment, such as leg braces, wheelchairs, and eating aids. These devices help patients perform daily tasks, allowing them to function more independently.

Some occupational therapists work with children in educational settings. They evaluate disabled children's abilities, modify classroom equipment to accommodate children with disabilities, and help children participate in school activities. Therapists also may provide early intervention therapy to infants and toddlers who have, or are at risk of having, developmental delays.

Therapists who work with older adults help their patients lead more independent and active lives. They assess patients' abilities and environments and make recommendations to improve the patients' everyday lives. For example, therapists may identify and recommend removal of potential fall hazards in a patient's home.

In some cases, occupational therapists help patients create functional work environments. They evaluate the workspace, recommend modifications, and meet with the patient's employer to collaborate on changes to the patient's work environment or schedule.

Occupational therapists also may work in mental health settings, where they help patients who suffer from developmental disabilities, mental illnesses, or emotional problems. Therapists teach these patients skills, such as managing time, budgeting, using public transportation, and doing household chores, to help them cope with and engage in daily life activities. In addition, therapists may work with individuals who have problems with drug abuse, alcoholism, depression, or other disorders. They may also work with people who have been through a traumatic event, such as a car accident.

Some occupational therapists, such as those employed in hospitals, work as part of a health care team along with doctors, registered nurses, and other types of therapists. They may work with patients who have chronic conditions, such as diabetes, or help rehabilitate patients recovering from hip replacement surgery. Occupational therapists also oversee the work of occupational therapy assistants and aides.

Public School Occupational Therapists

Following is a job description recruiting an occupational therapist in a public school system.

Sunshine Public Schools
Job Listing for
Occupational Therapist-1.0 FTE,
An Equal Opportunity Employer

SALARY $60,000 to $110,000 annually

OPENING DATE 01/01/20

CLOSING DATE 12/31/20

DESCRIPTION

Occupational therapists help students who have conditions that are mentally, physically, developmentally, or emotionally disabling improve their ability to perform tasks in daily routines and environments. They have the knowledge of treatments used to restore function that has been impaired or lost and improve the student's ability to perform tasks required for independent function. Specific occupational therapy services include but are not limited to: Using specifically designed activities and exercises to enhance neurodevelopmental, perceptual motor, sensory processing, and fine and gross motor functioning. They also help students develop, recover, or maintain daily living and school-based skills. They assist students in being able to access the educational environment. Occupational therapy services are federally mandated through the Individuals with Disabilities Education Act, governed by licensor laws, state administrative codes, and Individuals with Disabilities Education Act.

ESSENTIAL FUNCTIONS

1. Plans and implements treatment based upon evaluations and re-evaluations of eligible students (30% of time).
2. Evaluates, assesses, and observes and writes reports about findings for students as part of the multidisciplinary team evaluation for eligibility or for additional evaluation requests (20% of time).
3. Evaluates, assesses, and observes and writes reports for students as part of the multidisciplinary team re-evaluation process (10% of time).
4. Writes treatment plans—Individualized Education Programs—progress notes (10% of time).
5. Consults with teachers, parents, other staff members, and private-based medical professionals (5% of time).
6. Communicates via email or by phone with parents and private-based medical professionals (5% of time).

continued

7. Manages, operates, and makes minor repairs and adjustments to various equipment and supplies (5% of time).
8. Attends Individualized Education Program evaluation, staff, and other related meetings (5% of time).
9. Participates in education for students and provides program improvement recommendations (5% of time).
10. Performs related duties as appropriate to the assignment (5% of time).

   Conditions/Disclaimers: Employees may be required to perform duties outside of their normal responsibilities from time to time as needed. District employees are not authorized to make promises of employment for a particular period of time or promises of a particular level of compensation or benefits to job applicants for certified or classified positions, and that any such agreement must be in writing and signed by the superintendent. Any verbal or written statements to that effect by district employees other than the superintendent are null and void. Additionally, nothing in this job description restricts management's right to assign or reassign duties and responsibilities to this job at any time.

MINIMUM QUALIFICATIONS

Education

Bachelor's to master's degree in occupational therapy

Preferred: Bachelor's or master's degree in occupational therapy

Years of Experience

Will take new graduates

Preferred: Previous training and experience in pediatrics or school district

Certifications and Licenses

State Occupational Therapy License

Education Staff Associate certification

Continuing Education Training

Preferred: Training in school-based therapy or pediatric therapy methodology

Clearances

Criminal justice fingerprint or background check

Occupational Therapists in the Armed Services

- Air Force (https://www.airforce.com/careers/detail/occupational-therapist)
- Army (https://www.goarmy.com/careers-and-jobs/amedd-categories/medical-specialist-corps-jobs/occupational-therapist.html)
- Coast Guard (https://www.gocoastguard.com/active-duty-careers/officer-opportunities/programs/clinical-and-rehabilitation-therapist)
- Navy (https://www.navy.com/careers/occupational-therapy)

Following is a description of an occupational therapist in the U.S. Army, taken verbatim from the U.S. Army career site.

OVERVIEW

As a member of the Army Medical Specialist Corps, you will provide direct patient care, readiness training, wellness education, and injury prevention to our nation's soldiers. Occupational therapists have the opportunity to work in well-equipped U.S. Army medical centers and community hospitals, clinics, or field medical units.

JOB DUTIES

- Conduct battlefield unit needs assessments to determine unit mental health status.
- Conduct functional evaluations of and provide individualized treatment to soldiers suffering the effects of acute and chronic combat and operational stress.
- Serve as an independent practitioner and physician extender for acute and chronic upper extremity neuromuscular injuries and/or disorders, including the fabrication of custom splints to return injured soldiers to optimal duty status.
- Enhance unit and soldier performance by conducting energy conservation and work simplification assessments.
- Supervise enlisted and other qualified occupational therapy technicians implementing prescribed plans of care.
- Serve as commander of companies, battalions, brigades, and medical treatment facilities.
- Unique duty positions include: chief, Occupational Therapist Section, Specialist Corps; occupational therapy consultant; director, Occupational Therapy Military Unique Training Program

continued

REQUIREMENTS

Active Duty

- Bachelor's degree from an accredited occupational therapy program
- Completion of an occupational therapy field work experience
- Certification by the NBCOT
- Between 21 and 42 years of age
- U.S. citizenship
- Students graduating within 6 months, with a qualifying degree from a United States–accredited school, may apply for active U.S. Army service

Army Reserve

- In addition to the above qualifications, permanent United States residency and occupational therapy licensure are required for reserve duty officers.
- Between 21 and 42 years of age (may request a waiver, locate a recruiter for more information)

TRAINING

In the U.S. Army, the case diversity therapists experience in caring for soldiers far exceeds the medical care environment of the private sector. Our therapists work in well-equipped U.S. Army medical centers and Army community hospitals, clinics, and field medical units, and experience a wide range of practice environments.

During your tenure in the Army Medical Specialist Corps, you will have the unique opportunity to teach, become involved in research projects in your specialty, and work with people of all ages and backgrounds in support of community health and health education programs.

HELPFUL SKILLS

Army Medical Specialist Corps officers must be leaders skilled in tactics, techniques, and procedures to understand and support the soldier; possess strong Army values, leader attributes, and skills; and fully understand the key leadership actions that must be taken to ensure success.

Effective patient care requires the proper balance between technical skills and the ability to apply the appropriate treatment or procedure at the right moment. Army Medical Specialist Corps officers possess expert knowledge in their area of concentration, patient management, and general support and coordination principles. Therapists gain this knowledge through continuing medical education and experience sustained by mentoring, additional institutional training, continuous self-development and progressive levels of assignments within their specialty.

continued

COMPENSATION

Active Benefits

In addition to the many privileges that come with being an officer on the U.S. Army health care team, you'll be rewarded with:

- Specialty pay
- May receive pay for continuing education, including postgraduate training programs in orthopedics, emergency medicine, cardiopulmonary perfusion, and occupational medicine
- 30 days of paid vacation earned annually
- Noncontributory retirement benefits with 20 years of qualifying service
- No-cost or low-cost medical and dental care for you and your family

Reserve Benefits

- May receive pay for continuing education
- Noncontributory retirement benefits at age 60 with 20 years of qualifying service
- Travel opportunities, including humanitarian missions
- Low-cost dental and life insurance

Both active and reserve duty officers enjoy commissary and post exchange shopping privileges; a flexible, portable retirement savings and investment plan similar to a 401(k); and specialized training to become a leader in their field.

EARN CASH FOR IN-DEMAND JOBS

You could earn up to $40,000 in cash bonuses just for enlisting under certain Military Occupational Specialties. Visit Jobs in Demand (https://www.goarmy.com/home/jobs-in-demand.html) to see if this job qualifies for an enlistment bonus.

EDUCATION BENEFITS

As a member of the Army Medical Specialist Corps, you'll have access to the most sophisticated technologies, methods, and techniques in practice today; the opportunity to consult with experts in both the military and private sector; and exceptional professional growth opportunities, including continuing education courses, seminars, and conferences.

continued

FUTURE CIVILIAN CAREERS

As you advance through your career, you will be looking for experiences that blend teaching, research, and clinical excellence to best prepare you for unique and challenging opportunities. Our therapists excel in clinical, research, academic, and health administration arenas. Many have worked in more than one career track throughout their time in the Army and have held leadership positions ahead of their private sector counterparts. It's no surprise that U.S. Army therapists are highly desired candidates for competitive private sector jobs after their tenure with the Army Medical Specialist Corps.

PARTNERSHIP FOR YOUTH SUCCESS (PaYS) PROGRAM

Those interested in this job may be eligible for civilian employment, after the Army, by enrolling in the Army PaYS program. The PaYS program is a recruitment option that guarantees a job interview with military-friendly employers that are looking for experienced and trained veterans to join their organization. Find out more about the Army PaYS Program at http://www.armypays.com.

- Johns Hopkins
- GE Healthcare
- Cleveland Clinic
- Mercy Medical Center

Veterans Administration

There are also opportunities for occupational therapists to work in veterans administration hospitals and clinics. Below is a verbatim job description for an occupational therapist in a veterans administration hospital in Montana.

JOB DESCRIPTION

The staff occupational therapist will:

- Perform initial and ongoing assessments of the veteran's functional status.
- Evaluate the veteran's home for the structural modifications needed to make the home environment safe and accessible, and perform the initial and ongoing assessments of safety in the home environment.
- Determine the need for home medical equipment (HME).
- Teach and monitor the safe use of HME devices.

continued

- Report equipment problems to the Prosthetic and Sensory Aids Service.
- Teach body mechanics to the caregiver to minimize risk of injury.
- Establish a therapeutic program for the veteran and caregiver to maximize or maintain the veteran's functional status, and monitor the response.
- Supervise rehabilitation students assigned to the home-based primary care program.
- Collaborate with the veteran's primary care provider on patient needs for consultation with other rehabilitation services.

PRINCIPAL DUTIES AND RESPONSIBILITIES

- Uses knowledge of contemporary occupational therapy practice.
- Performs the initial and ongoing assessments of the veteran's functional status to determine extent of disability, including motor, sensory, integrative, activities of daily living, cognitive, perceptual, psychiatric, and present level of function using a full range of diagnostic tests and techniques, past, family, and social history, record review, and consultation with family and other health care practitioners.
- Exercises independent clinical judgment and adapts clinical procedures and techniques to accommodate age-specific and unique patient conditions, needs, and expectations.
- Consults with physicians and other health care practitioners related to diagnostic evaluation and treatment.
- Plans, coordinates, and implements a full range of patient-focused treatment services for veteran and caregiver designed to maximize or maintain the veteran's functional status, and monitoring the response.
- Evaluating the veteran's home for the structural modifications needed to make the home environment safe and accessible, and performing the initial and ongoing assessments of safety in the home environment.

WORK SCHEDULE

Monday through Friday; 8:00 am to 4:30 pm, or as agreed upon with the possibility of extended hours and weekends.

Note: Candidates must be willing to work weekends, irregular work hours, and extended hours. The candidate must be willing to be assigned to other related services and/or locations, if necessary.

FINANCIAL DISCLOSURE REPORT

Not required.

continued

BASIC REQUIREMENTS

United States Citizenship

Noncitizens may only be appointed when it is not possible to recruit qualified citizens in accordance with VA Policy.

Education

Graduation from a degree program in occupational therapy approved by the Accreditation Council for Occupational Therapy Education or predecessor organizations to include an internship (supervised field work experience required by the educational institution). The Accreditation Council for Occupational Therapy Education is the only accreditation agency recognized by the United States Department of Education and the Council for Higher Education Accreditation. Degree programs may be verified by contacting the American Occupational Therapy Association website or at their office address: American Occupational Therapy Association, P.O. Box 31220, Bethesda, MD 20824-1220.

Certification/Examination

Possession of written documentation that the individual has passed the entry-level certification examination for occupational therapists which is administered by the NBCOT.

English Language Proficiency

Occupational therapists must be proficient in spoken and written English in accordance with VA Handbook Part II, Chapter 3, Section A, Paragraph 3j.

Preferred: Experience with adaptive equipment and home modifications.

GRADE DETERMINATIONS

GS-11 Occupational Therapist

Education and Experience: In addition to meeting the basic requirements, completion of 1 year of progressively complex experience and a broader scope of experience equivalent to the next lower grade directly related to the position being filled, or 3 years of progressively higher level graduate education leading to a degree in occupational therapy or a directly related field.

Demonstrated Knowledge, Skills, Abilities and Other Characteristics: In addition to the basic requirements, individuals assigned as GS-11 occupational therapists must demonstrate all of the following knowledge, skills, abilities and other characteristics:

- Knowledge of advanced occupational therapy techniques to perform functions associated within the occupational therapy scope of practice
- Ability to communicate orally and in writing

continued

- Ability to adapt assessment tools and treatment to the complexity of the diagnosis or disabilities and demonstrate the clinical reasoning necessary to identify the need for further in-depth specific assessment of function and utilization of nonstandard methods and techniques
- Knowledge of principles and techniques in the occupational therapy assessment and treatment of occupational, cognitive, and psychological functional deficits

Reference: VA Handbook 5005/25, Part II, Appendix G14

PHYSICAL REQUIREMENTS

- Ability to spend approximately 75% of working day ambulating and standing
- Ability to frequently lift 60 pounds of force
- Ability to safely transfer patients and/or equipment using proper body mechanics (pushing, pulling, and lifting strategies)
- Ability to use the computer system

Important: A transcript must be submitted with your application if you are basing all or part of your qualifications on education.

Note: Only education or degrees recognized by the U.S. Department of Education from accredited colleges, universities, schools, or institutions may be used to qualify for federal employment. You can verify your education here: http://ope.ed.gov/accreditation/. If you are using foreign education to meet qualification requirements, you must send a Certificate of Foreign Equivalency with your transcript to receive credit for that education. For further information, visit: http://www.ed.gov/about/offices/list/ous/international/usnei/us/edlite-visitus-forrecog.html.

Job Outlook

Employment of occupational therapists is projected to grow 16% from 2019 to 2029, much faster than the average for all occupations. Occupational therapy will continue to be an important part of treatment for people with illnesses and disabilities, such as Alzheimer's disease, cerebral palsy, autism, or the loss of a limb.

For comparison, Table 2-2 provides current data and the occupational outlook for certified occupational therapy assistants, as detailed in the U.S. Bureau of Labor Statistics' *Occupational Outlook Handbook.*

TABLE 2-2. QUICK FACTS: OCCUPATIONAL THERAPY ASSISTANTS AND AIDES	
Median Pay, 2019	$59,200 per year $28.46 per hour
Work Experience in a Related Occupation	None
Number of Jobs, 2019	55,100
Job Outlook, 2019-2029	32% (Much faster than average)
Employment Change, 2019-2029	17,900
Reprinted from https://www.bls.gov/ooh	

WHAT DO OCCUPATIONAL THERAPY ASSISTANTS AND AIDES DO?

Occupational therapy assistants and aides help patients develop, recover, improve, as well as maintain the skills needed for daily living and working. Occupational therapy assistants are directly involved in providing therapy to patients; occupational therapy aides typically perform support activities. Both assistants and aides work under the direction of occupational therapists.

Work Environment

Occupational therapy assistants and aides work primarily in occupational therapists' offices, in hospitals, and in nursing care facilities. Occupational therapy assistants and aides spend much of their time on their feet while setting up equipment and, in the case of assistants, providing therapy to patients.

How to Become an Occupational Therapy Assistant or Aide

Occupational therapy assistants need an associate's degree from an accredited occupational therapy assistant program. All states regulate the practice of occupational therapy assistants. Occupational therapy aides typically need a high school diploma or equivalent and receive training on the job.

Job Outlook

Overall employment of occupational therapy assistants and aides is projected to grow 32% from 2019 to 2029, much faster than the average for all occupations. Occupational therapy will continue to be an important part of treatment for people with various illnesses and disabilities.

Learn more about occupational therapy assistants and aides by visiting additional resources, including O*NET, a source on key characteristics of workers and occupations.

Sample Job Description

Also included here for comparison is this job description for a certified occupational therapy assistant from PayScale (https://www.payscale.com/research/US/Job=Certified_Occupational_Therapy_Assistant_(COTA)/Hourly_Rate).

The position of certified occupational therapy assistant entails the oversight, administration, and assistance of occupational therapy activities. This position reports to and aids OTRs in applying therapies and occupational therapy techniques for the purpose of rehabilitation of people with injuries and/or disabilities. Rehabilitative services may be physical, emotional, psychological, or mental in nature, depending upon the need of the patients being served. Assistance and instruction directly to a patient and/or a patient's family may be required, so strong, professional, and interpersonal skills are preferred. Certified occupational therapy assistants must be able to document, organize, sort, and store information related to patient health, status, and progress, as well as billing, schedules, and other administrative documents and resources.

This job may involve physical assessment of patients and administration of therapies in health care settings, including clinical, outpatient, or home environments (this may involve driving to and from a patient's home to meet their needs). In-home and off-site work will often require direct supervision by an OTR but will sometimes include independent activity.

Background in physical therapy or applied kinesiology will be strongly beneficial. Certification must be assured for the completion of at least one of over 135 accredited occupational therapy assistant programs in the United States. Education requirements for this position will also involve at least an associate degree in a field directly related to occupational therapy. Compensation will be determined based on both the individual and the requirements of the occupational therapy firm. Individual compensation will be evaluated based on their certification, level of training, experience, and location.

SALARY AND BENEFITS FOR OCCUPATIONAL THERAPISTS

Job seekers usually focus on the salary offered and want the highest salary available. They do not necessarily take into consideration that salaries are not uniform across the country because the cost of living is not the same in all states. Salaries tend to be higher on the East and West coasts, where the cost of living is the highest. Salaries are a bit lower in the middle of the country. Also important is whether the salary is for 9, 10, 11, or 12 months, or is being quoted as an hourly salary for part-time (fewer than 40 hours per week) or full-time (40 hours per week). Salaries for private and public school positions are often quoted for 9 or 10 months because the school year is 9 or 10 months, not 12 months, long. College and university salaries may also be quoted for 9 or 10 months. If a summer session is available but optional, the quote may be for 11 months. Most hospital, clinic, or nursing home salaries are quoted for 12 months.

For example, imagine a job at Sunnyside School is quoted in an advertisement for $60,000, and another advertisement for the Metropolitan Hospital is quoted at $80,000. The hospital position appears to be paying a much better salary—until the different base is examined. When the school salary is prorated from 9 to 12 months, both salaries are the same. For practitioners with children, the school position may be a better option since both parent and children would be free from school and work activities at the same time during the summer months. A 12-month position might require child care expenses unless a relative or friend is willing to provide free child care services.

Other considerations are the travel expenses to and from the job. A higher paycheck can quickly be reduced if the distance to the workplace takes an hour or more and parking a vehicle requires a parking fee. The cost of gas, parking, and increased maintenance on the vehicle may outweigh the higher salary. If time is also considered, the increased time to commute to work should be factored into the equation. More travel time means less recreation and relaxation time. Another factor is stress. Longer commutes tend to be more stressful. A better quality of life may be more important than a higher paycheck. Of course, another stress factor is paying off the student loan debt. Deciding on which stress factors to endure may determine the place of employment.

In addition to salary, the employee benefit or compensation package should be examined. A good benefit package may be more useful than a higher salary. Benefit packages may include medical and dental insurance, disability or worker's compensation insurance, sick leave, retirement and pension plans, paid vacation, paid family or medical leave, paid child care, paid or subsidized parking, tuition and time off to attend college classes, travel assistance or reimbursement for continuing education expenses, free or subsidized meals, housing and moving assistance, discounts on selected services or products such as membership in a fitness club, use of a company vehicle, end-of-year bonus, and stock options or profit-sharing.

Some types of employee benefits are mandated by law for organizations that employ 500 or more employees. These include minimum wage, payment for overtime. leave-of-absence time under the Family Medical Leave Act, unemployment insurance, and workers' compensation and disability insurance.

Salaries for occupational therapy practitioners are higher than the minimum wage, so that benefit is guaranteed. The arrangement for overtime pay depends on the type of payment schedule; employees paid on an hourly basis are eligible for overtime pay, while those paid per week or by the month are not, because they are paid to perform stated job duties and to organize their time and effort accordingly. The other mandated benefits usually do apply to occupational therapy practitioner positions in larger institutions.

All of the other items are considered fringe benefits or perks. Employers can offer as many as they wish, or none at all. Therefore, the job seeker must ask which are available, and may be able to negotiate for additional benefits or trade one benefit for another. Some employers provide what is often called a *cafeteria plan*. Each employee is allotted a set amount of money and allowed to select the most personally important items from the benefit list within the monetary cap or other limit set by the employer. The advantage of the cafeteria plan is that the potential employee picks the benefits of greatest value or usefulness, as opposed to a fixed benefit package applied to all employees whether they benefit from the services or not. For example, for an employee who drives to work, a paid parking benefit is useful, but for the employee who rides the bus to work, the benefit is useless.

If a cafeteria plan is not available, the job seeker may be able to negotiate for a benefit package that better suits individual needs. For example, if paid parking is provided but the potential employee rides a bus, the candidate could ask if the paid parking option could be traded for tuition and travel assistance, or reimbursement to attend continuing education activities required to maintain a state license. Both the employee and employer may benefit from such an arrangement. The cost of attending continuing education activities is reduced for the employee, and the employer has helped ensure that the employee maintains a license to practice. Another option may be to forgo all the fringe benefits not required by law and negotiate for a higher salary. For example, if an employee has medical insurance under a family plan provided by the spouse, this expensive benefit for the employer may be a bargaining chip for the employee to offer in a bid for a higher salary or other more useful benefits.

All these examples assume that a benefit package is available and that choices can be made. In some cases, the only benefits available are those required by law. School-based positions, for example, usually do not offer paid vacation because the position only covers 9 months, leaving 3 months free for vacation or other paid positions depending on the individual's choice. The same school-based position may not offer tuition assistance for continuing education because professional enhancement days are built into the school calendar for all teachers and other professional-level employees.

In summary, when searching for a job as an occupational therapy practitioner, be sure to look beyond the salary figure to examine the benefit package. If the information is not provided, ask for and examine the details, weigh any options, select the best choices, then negotiate to get the salary figure and benefits package that best suit your needs.

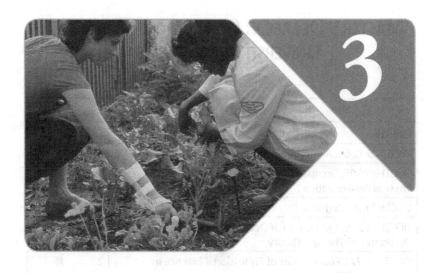

3

Typical Curriculums for
Master's and Associate Degrees
in Occupational Therapy

Stein, F., & Reed, K. L.
*Occupational Therapy: A Guide for Prospective
Students, Consumers, and Advocates* (pp. 29-42).
© 2021 Taylor & Francis Group.

MASTER'S DEGREE IN OCCUPATIONAL THERAPY— UNIVERSITY OF WISCONSIN

YEAR 1: FALL	
COURSE	**CREDITS**
PRPP 725: Gross Anatomical Kinesiology	3
OCCTHPY 705: Occupational Therapy in Physical Rehabilitation I	3
OCCTHPY 707: Seminar I	1
OCCTHPY 720: Application of Occupational Science and Occupational Therapy Theory	3
OCCTHPY 721: Foundations of Professional Practice in Occupational Therapy	2
OCCTHPY 880: Master's Project	1
1st Level I Fieldwork (January-April)	
TOTAL CREDITS	*13*
YEAR 1: SPRING	
COURSE	**CREDITS**
OCCTHPY 703: Applied Neuroscience	3
OCCTHPY 704: Musculoskeletal Analysis and Occupational Function	3
OCCTHPY 706: Occupational Therapy in Physical Rehabilitation II (Part 1)	2
OCCTHPY 708: Seminar II	1
OCCTHPY 740: Occupational Therapy With Children and Families	4
OCCTHPY 880: Master's Project	1
2nd Level I Fieldwork (after summer courses—August, or third semester—Fall)	
TOTAL CREDITS	*14*

Reprinted with permission from University of Wisconsin.

YEAR 1: SUMMER	
COURSE	**CREDITS**
OCCTHPY 540: Evidence for Practice I	3
OCCTHPY 706: Occupational Therapy in Physical Rehabilitation II (Part 2)	3
OCCTHPY 719: Occupational Therapy in Psychosocial Practice	3
Optional Electives/Thesis	
2nd Level I Fieldwork (after summer courses—August, or third semester—Fall)	
TOTAL CREDITS	*9*

YEAR 2: FALL	
COURSE	**CREDITS**
OCCTHPY 519: Therapeutic Communication	3
OCCTHPY 542: Evidence for Practice II	3
OCCTHPY 620: Introduction to Assistive Technology and Rehabilitation Technologies U/G	3
OCCTHPY 709: Seminar III	1
OCCTHPY 880: Master's Project	1
Required Electives/Thesis	3
2nd Level I Fieldwork (September-November, unless completed in Summer)	
TOTAL CREDITS	*14*

Reprinted with permission from University of Wisconsin.

YEAR 2: SPRING

COURSE	CREDITS
• OCCTHPY 725: Occupational Therapy Field Service I (off-campus January-March)	6
Optional Electives for Early Spring: OCCTHPY 718: Occupational Therapy in Acute Care OCCTHPY 743: Advances in Child-Centered Occupational Therapy	0
OCCTHPY 744: Advanced Occupational Therapy for Aging Adults	3
TOTAL CREDITS	9

YEAR 2: SUMMER

COURSE	CREDITS
OCCTHPY 710: Commmunication Models of Occupational Therapy Practice	2
OCCTHPY 711: Professional Leadership of Occupational Therapists	3
Optional Elective/Thesis	
TOTAL CREDITS	5

YEAR 3: FALL

COURSE	CREDITS
OCCTHPY 735: Occupational Therapy Field Service II (off-campus October-December)	6
OCCTHPY 810: Critical Evaluation of Theory, Research, and Practice (3 weeks)	2
Optional Elective	
TOTAL CREDITS	8

Reprinted with permission from University of Wisconsin.

TYPICAL ENTRY-LEVEL ASSOCIATE DEGREE CURRICULUM FOR A CERTIFIED OCCUPATIONAL THERAPY ASSISTANT (SMITH TECHNICAL COLLEGE [STC])

OCCUPATIONAL THERAPY ASSISTANT (2019-2020)

Associate in Applied Science Degree

School of Health Sciences

PROGRAM CODE 10-555-5

TELEPHONE 555-555-1234

OVERVIEW

This program prepares you to become a certified occupational therapy assistant.

In the traditional setting, the certified occupational therapy assistant provides services under the supervision of an occupational therapist using goal-directed activities to prevent, lessen, or overcome difficulty in attaining, maintaining, or developing occupations: daily living, play, leisure, and/or work skills. Services are provided in various environments, including hospitals, geriatric centers, schools, and homes.

A health care provider cardiopulmonary resuscitation certificate is a prerequisite for entry into the fourth clinical course. Note that the occupational therapy assistant program must be completed within 4 years.

ACCREDITATION INFORMATION

Accreditation Council for Occupational Therapy Education; www.acoteonline.org

CAREER PATHWAY

This program features exploratory courses that count toward a credential.

CAREER OUTLOOK

The certified occupational therapy assistant can look forward to a positive job outlook. Opportunities can be found in hospitals, rehabilitation centers, geriatric centers, schools, and homes. Employment includes working with persons experiencing developmental disabilities, mental illness, physical disabilities, and the results of aging. For additional career information, visit www.promoteot.org.

continued

PROGRAM LEARNING OUTCOMES

- Demonstrate professional behaviors, ethical standards, values, and attitudes of the occupational therapy profession
- Practice within the distinct role and responsibility of the certified occupational therapy assistant
- Advocate for the profession, services, and consumers
- Value lifelong learning and the need to keep current with best practice
- Apply occupational therapy principles and intervention tools to achieve expected outcomes
- Serve a diverse population in a variety of systems that are consistent with entry-level practice

ADMISSION REQUIREMENTS

This program admits students through a petition selection process.

Learn more about the petition process.

HP-A2 HESI Preadmission exam required.

The following are also required for admission:

- A high school diploma or GED
- One year of high school–level or one semester of college-level algebra, biology, and chemistry; with a grade of C or higher for each course
- Demonstration of proficiency in basic skills through a course placement assessment

This program's required natural science courses must be completed with a grade of B- or higher in each course.

POSSIBLE CAREERS

Certified Occupational Therapy Assistant

Occupational Therapy Assistant

RELATED PROGRAMS

Physical Therapist Assistant

Registered Nurse

Respiratory Therapist

continued

START DATE

August

16-week terms

This program will transfer to one or more 4-year institutions.

Program curriculum requirements are subject to change.

For course descriptions, times, visit website for course descriptions, times, locations, and registration.

Students who have not been accepted, or have not decided on a program, may begin with General Studies courses, if course prerequisites have been met.

TECHNICAL STUDIES			CREDITS
( ) = Semester Order for Full-Time Students			
(1)	OTASST-171	Introduction to Occupational Therapy ‡	3
(1)	OTASST-172	Medical and Psychosocial Conditions # ‡	3
(1)	OTASST-173	Activity Analysis and Application ‡	2
(2)	OTASST-174	Occupational Therapy Performance Skills ‡	4
(2)	OTASST-176	Occupational Therapy Theory and Practice ‡	3
(2)	OTASST-177	Assistive Technology and Adaptations ‡	2
(2)	OTASST-178	Geriatric Practice ‡	3
(3)	OTASST-175	Psychosocial Practice ‡	3
(3)	OTASST-179	Community Practice ‡	2
(3)	OTASST-182	Physical Rehabilitation Practice ‡	3
(3)	OTASST-183	Pediatric Practice ‡	3
(3)	OTASST-184	Occupational Therapy Assistant Fieldwork ‡	2
(4)	OTASST-185	Occupational Therapy Practice and Management # ‡	2
(4)	OTASST-186	Occupational Therapy Assistant Fieldwork 2A * ‡	5
(4)	OTASST-187	Occupational Therapy Assistant Fieldwork 2B * ‡	5

GENERAL STUDIES		CREDITS
ENG-151	Communication Skills 1 ‡	3
and ENG-152	Communication Skills 2 ‡ (or) ENG-201 ‡ and any 200-series ENG or SPEECH course	3
NATSCI-177	General Anatomy and Physiology ‡ (or) NATSCI-201 Anatomy and Physiology 1 ‡ and NATSCI-202 Anatomy and Physiology 2 ‡	4
PSYCH-159	Abnormal Psychology (or) PSYCH-232 Abnormal Psychology ‡	3
PSYCH-188	Developmental Psychology (or) PSYCH-238 Lifespan Psychology	3
PSYCH-199	Psychology of Human Relations (or) PSYCH-231 Introductory Psychology	3
SOCSCI-172	Introduction to Diversity Studies (or) Any 200-series HIST or SOCSCI course	3
ELECTIVES	Suggested Electives: Three Credits Needed	3
HEALTH-101	Medical Terminology	
PHYED-210	An Active Approach to Wellness and Fitness	
SOCSCI-210	Death and Dying	
TOTAL CREDITS		70
# OTASST-172 and OTASST-185 are online courses.		
* OTASST-186 and OTASST-187 must be completed within 18 months following academic coursework.		
‡ Prerequisite required.		

What Are the Similarities and Differences Between a Registered Occupational Therapist and a Certified Occupational Therapy Assistant?

According to Top Occupational Therapy Schools, the following summary highlights similarities and differences between the professionals of occupational therapist and occupational therapy assistant.

Skills and Qualities

Occupational Therapist

Skills and qualities that an occupational therapist must have are as follows:

- Extraordinary leadership qualities
- Good writing skills
- Excellent communication skills
- Compassion and interpersonal skills
- Operation analyzing abilities
- Capability to identify indicators of system performance
- Should be a good instructor
- Complex problem-solving abilities
- Time management skills
- Good natured and cooperative attitude
- Adaptability and flexibility
- Persistent and innovative
- Highly responsible and autonomous

Occupational Therapy Assistant

A good occupational therapy assistant must possess these traits and abilities:

- Good communication skills
- Good physical strength
- Digital skills to operate equipment and devices
- Great teamworking skills to collaborate with the team members and other professionals
- Excellent writing skills to keep records of the clients
- Social perceptiveness
- Time managing skills
- Should be an active listener

- Problem sensitivity
- Compassion and interpersonal skills
- Information-gathering abilities
- Critical thinking skills
- Interested in promoting health and well-being

Responsibilities

Occupational Therapist

Being an occupational therapist, individuals have to undertake the following responsibilities and duties:

- Teach anxiety management tricks and techniques
- Guide people to return to workplace
- Teach people to control their behavior
- Provide program to the students
- Supervise occupational therapy assistants and aides
- Organize rehabilitation and support groups for patients and careers
- Set up a rehabilitation program to rebuild lost skills and regain confidence
- Instruct on home and office environmental adjustments, for instance, alterations in the use of wheelchair
- Coach to use specialist equipment to assist people suffering problems in day-to-day activities
- Guide people who face problems in learning or the ones who have poor social skills
- Communicate with other team members and professionals, such as doctors, occupational therapists, architects, equipment dealers, suppliers, patient's family members, guardians, and employers
- Prepare a caseload, analyze patient's priorities, requirements, and needs
- Do administrative tasks, such as budgetary records
- Evaluate and analyze the evaluation data, such as interpretation of records contributed by an occupational therapy assistant
- Write and sign assessment report for the evaluation team report
- Develop and modify the plan of care in collaboration with the occupational therapy assistant and decide which part of the plan will be implemented by the occupational therapy assistant
- Direct occupational therapy assistants and aides, take their periodic inspection, collaborate with them, and provide in-service programs to them

- Review, revise, and cosign the occupational therapy assistants' daily notes and treatments
- Do proper analysis for periodic revision and collaborate with the individualized education program (IEP) team and the occupational therapy assistant to determine new aims and objectives and decide if therapies should be continued or not
- Write discharge summary and plan when services are terminated

Occupational Therapy Assistant

Responsibilities of an occupational therapy assistant are as follows:

- Assist patients with poor social skills and learning disabilities
- Help the patients to carry out their routine activities and tasks
- Analyze patients' activities to know whether they are done properly or not
- Handle administrative as well as clerical tasks
- Teach patients the correct way to use special devices and equipment that are essential for their daily activities
- Give regular reports about patient to occupational therapists
- Work to help disabled children and aid them in playing activities and games that can augment their skills and abilities
- Work under occupational therapists and plan rehabilitation programs
- Refer requests for all the services of occupational therapy to occupational therapists
- Participate in the evaluation process by accumulating data, managing standardized tests or objective measurement, and reporting observations
- Assist occupational therapists and IEP to achieve the goals and targets of IEP
- Participate and collaborate in the preparation, implementation, and documentation of the occupational therapy intervention plan. They are independent to choose treatment activities and tasks as per the occupational therapy intervention plan.
- Document intervention or therapy sessions and outcomes and discuss with an occupational therapist regarding students' needs, progress, and intervention plan
- Properly prepare periodic progress reports to be reviewed and cosigned by an occupational therapist
- Keep an eye on whether the occupational therapist cosigns and reviews daily reports about the patient or not

- Give data for assessment to occupational therapist and IEP and participate with them for periodic review of all the reports
- Give all the necessary details and information to an occupational therapist and assist in forming a discharge plan at the time of termination of occupational therapy services

Adapted from https://www.topoccupationaltherapyschool.com/ot-vs-ota-difference/

COSTS FOR OCCUPATIONAL THERAPY STUDENTS

According to CostHelper Education (https://www.education.costhelper. com/occupational-therapist.html), the following information details what it costs to become an occupational therapist.

A master's degree in occupational therapy typically costs $15,000 to $70,000. For example, Milligan College, a private college in Tennessee, offers the 79-credit master's degree in occupational therapy for $49,000. A public school, the University of New Mexico offers a master's degree in occupational therapy from $15,000 for state residents taking the maximum number of courses per semester, to $70,000 for nonresidents taking courses at a slower pace.

There are only a handful of accredited doctorate programs in occupational therapy, costing $43,000 to $108,000 and typically taking 3 to 5 years to complete. Washington University in St. Louis, Missouri, estimates tuition costs of $108,000 over 5 years for their occupational therapy doctorate program. The University of Toledo in Ohio estimates tuition of $42,800 for Ohio residents or $81,200 for nonresidents over the eight-semester doctorate program. The occupational therapy doctorate program at Belmont University in Nashville, Tennessee, costs $99,800 over seven semesters.

Board certification costs $500 and can be earned by taking the exam with the National Board for Certification in Occupational Therapy, which meets the requirements to practice as an occupational therapist in most states. After passing the test, practitioners can use the title "Occupational Therapist Registered."

State licensing fees are typically $90 to $300. Washington's occupational therapist licensing fee is $175, while New York's fee is $294. All states require registration or licensure to practice occupational therapy, and links to state licensing boards can be found at the California Board of Occupational Therapy.

SCHOLARSHIPS FOR
OCCUPATIONAL THERAPY STUDENTS

Many opportunities for scholarships are available from the American Occupational Therapy Association, state and local agencies, and private foundations.

CollegeScholarships.com is valuable in identifying a scholarship in a specific category (https://www.collegescholarships.com/major-degree/occupational-therapy-scholarships).

- Scholarships by major
- Scholarships by state
- Local scholarships
- Scholarships for women
- Scholarship of the month
- Religious scholarships
- Sports scholarships
- Military scholarships
- Disability scholarships
- Unusual scholarships
- Financial aid
- Scholarship essay examples

Top Occupational Therapy Schools also has links to occupational therapy education scholarships (https://www.topoccupationaltherapyschool.com/scholarships-grants-occupational-therapists/).

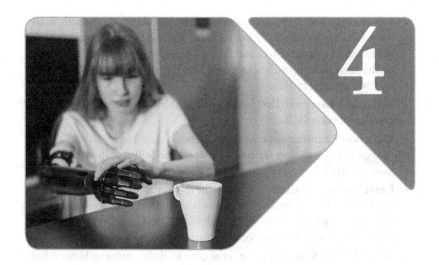

Comparing
Occupational Therapy to
Similar Health Professions

OTHER HEALTH PROFESSIONS

Activity Therapist

- **Educational Requirements:** Varies from high school diploma to master's degree depending on the level of certification sought or requirements of other single modality therapy services, such as recreation, music, art, or dance.
- **Professional Organization:** National Certification Council for Activity Professionals.

Stein, F., & Reed, K. L.
Occupational Therapy: A Guide for Prospective
Students, Consumers, and Advocates (pp. 43-56).
© 2021 Taylor & Francis Group.

- **Job Description:** Develop, coordinate, and evaluate therapeutic activity programs for clients. May include conducting sports and exercise activities, conducting arts and crafts classes, organizing trips to events in the community, or developing a schedule of social activities within and without the facility.
- **Personal Characteristics:** Interpersonal skills, and verbal and written communication skills.
- **Licensure Requirements:** No state license is required for title of activity therapist, but a person trained in a single modality, such as recreation, may require a license in some states.
- **Certification:** Available through the National Certification Council for Activity Professionals. Three levels: Activity Professional Certified, Activity Director Certified, and Activity Consultant Certified. Certification may or may not be required at a given work setting.
- **Typical Work Settings:** Long-term care facilities, nursing homes, hospitals with rehabilitation programs, behavioral health programs.
- **Salary Range:** $35,000 to $50,000 per year.

Art Therapist

- **Educational Requirements:** Master's degree in art education or art therapy with courses in human development, psychological and behavioral disorders, counseling theory, and therapeutic techniques.
- **Professional Organization:** American Art Therapy Association.
- **Job Description:** Art therapy uses the creative process of art as a form of expressive therapy to facilitate the process of helping clients to explore their feelings, understand their emotional conflicts, develop social skills, improve self-esteem, reduce anxiety, and restore normal function in their lives.
- **Personal Characteristics:** Interest in and appreciation of the visual arts and forms, such as sculpture, painting, drawing, or illustration and experience in a variety of art mediums. Skills in creativity, critical thinking, interpersonal interaction, organization, and communication are important.
- **Licensure Requirements:** Usually in psychology or counseling.
- **Certification:** Available from the Art Therapy Credentials Board.
- **Typical Work Settings:** Hospitals, rehabilitation care units, assisted living centers, psychiatric facilities, senior communities, schools, or private practice.
- **Salary Range:** $50,000 to $70,000 per year.

Athletic Trainer

- **Educational Requirements:** Bachelor's degree or higher.
- **Professional Organization:** National Athletic Trainers' Association.
- **Job Description:** Athletic trainers prevent, diagnose, and treat muscle and bone injuries and illnesses.
- **Personal Characteristics:** Interpersonal skills, verbal and written communication skills, teaching and instructing skills, concern for others, practical, adaptability, mental flexibility, dependable, and stress tolerance.
- **Licensure Requirements:** Requirements for license or certification vary by state.
- **Certification:** Available through the Board of Certification for the Athletic Trainer.
- **Typical Work Settings:** Most athletic trainers work in educational settings, such as colleges, universities, and public or private schools. Others work in hospitals, fitness centers, physicians' offices, or for professional sports teams.
- **Salary Range:** $45,000 to $60,000.

Audiologist

- **Educational Requirements:** Doctoral degree in audiology.
- **Professional Organization:** American Academy of Audiology.
- **Job Description:** Audiologists diagnose, manage, and treat clients with hearing, balance or other ear- or hearing-related problems.
- **Personal Characteristics:** Interpersonal skills, communication skills, teaching and instructing skills, concern for others, investigative using facts and figuring out problems, cooperative with others, attention to detail, honest and ethical, and dependable.
- **Licensure Requirements:** License required in all states, but specific requirements vary by state.
- **Certification:** Available through the American Speech-Language-Hearing Association (Certificate of Clinical Competence).
- **Typical Work Settings:** Audiologists work in physicians' offices, audiology clinics, hospitals, private and public schools, private practice settings, and businesses that sell hearing aids and services.
- **Salary Range:** $75,000 to $90,000.

Child Life Specialist

- **Educational Requirements:** Bachelor's or master's degree in a field of study, such as psychology, human growth and development, education, or counseling, plus a national examination and 480 hours of clinical internship under a certified child life specialist.
- **Professional Organization:** Association of Child Life Professionals.
- **Job Description:** Child life specialists use their knowledge to explain procures and medical terminology at the level appropriate to the child's development and understanding, to provide emotional support to children and parents or caregivers during procedures, and to teach the child skills to cope with the stress and anxiety throughout with issues related to the disorder or illness.
- **Personal Characteristics:** Concern for others, interpersonal skills, teaching and instructing skills, patience and tolerance, and interest in children.
- **Licensure Requirements:** See Certification.
- **Certification:** The certification examination is administered through the Association of Child Life Professionals.
- **Typical Work Settings:** Hospitals with large pediatric departments.
- **Salary Range:** $40,000 to $55,000.

Creative Arts Therapist (Expressive Art Therapist)

- **Educational Requirements:** Usually a master's degree, but each art form has its own requirements.
- **Professional Organization:** National Coalition of Creative Arts Therapies Association.
- **Job Description:** Creative arts therapists help individuals, families, and groups to improve their overall physical and mental health by applying the principles and techniques of each art form to improve communications, allow expression of feelings, improve coordination, and increase cognitive and social function. Most creative arts therapists specialize in a single area, such as art, dance and movement, drama, music, or poetry.
- **Personal Characteristics:** Skill in the focused art form or forms. Research each art form for additional characteristics.
- **Licensure Requirements:** May require a state license depending on the state and chosen art form or forms.

- **Certification:** A program of certification is available for most art forms. The national organization is called the National Organization for Arts in Health.

- **Typical Work Settings:** Hospitals, nursing homes, rehabilitation clinics and facilities, correctional institutions, halfway houses, residential treatment centers, behavioral health centers, and art studios.

- **Salary Range:** $35,000 to $70,000.

Dance Therapist/Movement Therapist

- **Educational Requirements:** Master's degree from a program approved by the American Dance Therapy Association (ADTA).

- **Professional Organization:** ADTA.

- **Job Description:** Dance/movement therapy uses dance and movement to promote social, cognitive, and physical health and wellness in clients.

- **Personal Characteristics:** Compassion, patience, empathy, physical fitness, knowledge of and skill in a variety of types of dances.

- **Licensure Requirements:** Some states require a license in psychology or counseling.

- **Certification:** Registration with the ADTA (entry-level) or board certification with ADTA (advanced).

- **Typical Work Settings:** Psychiatric hospitals, rehabilitation centers, drug treatment facilities, counseling and crisis centers, and private dance studios.

- **Salary Range:** $60,000 to $70,000 per year.

Kinesiotherapist

- **Educational Requirements:** Bachelor's degree or higher from a program in kinesiotherapy accredited by the Commission on Accreditation of Allied Health Education Programs.

- **Professional Organization:** American Kinesiotherapy Association.

- **Job Description:** Kinesiotherapists develop and monitor exercise programs to help clients regain muscle strength and function loss due to disease or injury.

- **Personal Characteristics:** Adaptability, good interpersonal skills, patience, good sense of humor, good in science (e.g., anatomy, physiology, physics), and good communication skills.

- **Licensure Requirements:** None.

- **Certification:** Registration examination administered by the Council on Professional Standards for Kinesiotherapy Registration Board.

- **Typical Work Settings:** Veteran's facilities, hospitals, clinics, and home care.
- **Salary Range:** $60,000 to $80,000 per year.

Music Therapist

- **Educational Requirements:** Bachelor's degree or higher in an approved music therapy program.
- **Professional Organization:** American Music Therapy Association.
- **Job Description:** Music therapists assess emotional well-being, physical health, social functioning, communication abilities, and cognitive skills through musical responses; design music sessions for individuals and groups based on client needs using music improvisation, receptive music listening, song writing, lyric discussion, music and imagery, musical performance, and learning through music.
- **Personal Characteristics:** Accomplished musician, versatile, patient, empathetic, imaginative, tactful, sense of humor and creativity, openness to new ideas, skills in oral and written communication, and ability to work well with other health care providers.
- **Licensure Requirements:** Some states require a license in psychology or counseling.
- **Certification:** Board certification through the Certification Board for Music Therapists.
- **Typical Work Settings:** Psychiatric hospitals, rehabilitation facilities, mental health facilities, outpatient clinics, day care treatment centers, nursing homes, hospice programs, correctional facilities, halfway houses, schools, and private practice.
- **Salary Range:** $40,000 to $60,000 per year.

Physical Therapist

- **Educational Requirements:** Doctoral degree in physical therapy.
- **Professional Organization:** American Physical Therapy Association.
- **Job Description:** Physical therapists help clients with injuries or diseases improve their movement and manage their pain.
- **Personal Characteristics:** Interpersonal skills, concern for others, oral and written communication, teaching and instructing skills, investigative skills using facts and figuring out problems, practical, self-controlled, dependable, honest, and ethical.
- **Licensure Requirements:** Physical therapists are licensed in all 50 states.

- **Typical Work Settings:** Private practice, hospitals, clinics, nursing homes, and home care.
- **Salary Range:** $80,000 to $100,000.

Psychologist

- **Educational Requirements:** Doctoral degree.
- **Professional Organization:** American Psychological Association, National Association of School Psychologists, American School Counselor Association, American Counseling Association.
- **Job Description:** Psychologists study cognitive, emotional, and social processes and behavior by observing, interpreting, and recording how individuals relate to one another and to their environment. They use their findings to facilitate improvement in behavior and processes.
- **Personal Characteristics:** Interpersonal skills, communication skills, teaching and instructing skills, investigative skills using facts and figuring out problems, working without a clear set of rules, concern for others, self-controlled, socially oriented, dependable, honest, and ethical.
- **Licensure Requirements:** All states require a license to practice. The specific license depends on the type of specialization within the field of psychology, such as school psychology, clinical psychology, or counseling psychology.
- **Certification:** Specialized certification is available with the American Board for Professional Psychology.
- **Typical Work Settings:** Public and private schools, hospitals, clinics, mental health facilities, correctional institutions, private practice.
- **Salary Range:** $75,000 to $90,000.

Recreation Therapist
(Certified Therapeutic Recreation Specialist)

- **Educational Requirements:** Bachelor's degree in recreational therapy or related field, such as recreation and leisure studies with an emphasis on therapeutic recreation.
- **Professional Organization:** American Therapeutic Recreation Association.
- **Job Description:** Recreation therapists plan, direct, and coordinate recreation-based treatment for clients with disabilities, injuries, or illnesses. They use a variety of modalities, including arts and crafts, drama, music, dance, sports, games, aquatics, and community outings, to help clients maintain or improve physical, social, and emotional well-being.

- **Personal Characteristics:** Interpersonal skills, communication skills, listening skills, teaching and instructing skills, leadership skills, adaptability, mental flexibility, integrity, concern for others, cooperative with others, dependable, honest and ethical, compassionate, resourceful, and patient.
- **Licensure Requirements:** Some states, but not all, require a license.
- **Certification:** The certification program is maintained by the National Council for Therapeutic Recreation Certification.
- **Typical Work Settings:** Hospitals, residential facilities, community mental health centers, adult day care programs, substance abuse centers, hospice care, community centers, school systems, and private practice.
- **Salary Range:** $50,000 to $60,000.

Rehabilitation Counselor
(Vocational Rehabilitation Counselor)

- **Educational Requirements:** Master's degree in vocational counseling, rehabilitation counseling, or psychology counseling.
- **Professional Organization:** American Rehabilitation Counseling Association.
- **Job Description:** Vocational rehabilitation counselors help clients with disabilities live fuller, more independent lives by assisting them to secure gainful employment. They assess clients' capabilities and limitations, help clients set employment goals, facilitate job training and placement, assist in job application processes, provide mock interviews, and advocate for employment of people with disabilities.
- **Personal Characteristics:** Interpersonal skills, communication skills, teaching and instructing skills, concern for others, investigative skills using facts and figuring out problems, cooperative, honest and ethical, dependable, and self-control.
- **Licensure Requirements:** State license is a licensed professional counselor.
- **Certification:** The certification program is maintained by the Commission on Rehabilitation Counselor Certification and includes an examination.
- **Typical Work Settings:** Community rehabilitation centers, youth guidance organization, and senior citizen centers.
- **Salary Range:** $30,000 to $50,000.

Special Education Teacher

- **Educational Requirements:** Bachelor's degree or higher.
- **Professional Organization:** National Association of Special Education Teachers.
- **Job Description:** Special education teachers work with students who have a wide range of learning, mental, emotional, and physical disabilities. They adapt general education lessons and teach various subjects, such as reading, writing, and math, to students with mild and moderate disabilities. They also teach basic skills, such as literacy and communication techniques, to students with severe disabilities.
- **Personal Characteristics:** Teaching and instructing skills, verbal and written communication, interpersonal skills, concern for others, adaptability, mental flexibility, honest and ethical, cooperative with others, dependable, good self-control, and ability to function without a clear set of rules.
- **Licensure Requirements:** All states require a teaching certificate or license and may have additional requirements for teachers of special education.
- **Typical Work Settings:** Most special education teachers work in public schools, teaching students from preschool to high school. Other work settings include private schools, child care services, hospitals, and state institutions.
- **Salary Range:** $45,000 to $70,000.

Social Worker, Clinical

- **Educational Requirements:** Master's degree or higher.
- **Professional Organization:** National Association of Social Workers.
- **Job Description:** Social workers help people solve and cope with problems in their everyday lives. Clinical social workers also diagnose and treat mental, behavioral, and emotional issues.
- **Personal Characteristics:** Interpersonal skills, communication skills, teaching and instructing skills, investigative skills using facts and figuring out problems, concern for others, cooperative with others, honest and ethical, dependable, and stress tolerant.
- **Licensure Requirements:** Required for clinical social workers.
- **Certification:** Specialty certification is available through the National Association of Social Workers.

- **Typical Work Settings:** Mental health clinics, public and private schools, child welfare and human service agencies, hospitals, clinics, community development centers, and private practice.
- **Salary Range:** $50,000 to $70,000.

Speech-Language Pathologist (Speech Therapist)

- **Educational Requirements:** Master's degree or higher in speech-language pathology.
- **Professional Organization:** American Speech-Language Hearing Association.
- **Job Description:** Speech-language pathologists assess, diagnose, treat, and help to prevent communication and swallowing disorders in children and adults.
- **Personal Characteristics:** Interpersonal skills, concern for others, oral and written communication, teaching and instructing others, adaptability, mental flexibility, cooperative with others, dependable, and honest.
- **Licensure Requirements:** Most states require speech-language pathologists to be licensed.
- **Certification:** Available through the American Speech-Language Hearing Association (Certificate of Clinical Competence).
- **Typical Work Settings:** Public and private schools, hospitals, clinics, and private practice.
- **Salary Range:** $75,000 to $95,000.

Note: Salaries are general based on 2017 to 2018 data and may vary by location or facility.
https://www.bls.gov/ooh/

WITH WHOM DO OCCUPATIONAL THERAPISTS AND ASSISTANTS WORK?

Depending on the type and location of the occupational therapy position, a variety of other professionals, colleagues, and coworkers may be team members. The list below provides a brief description of some of the team members, their roles, and qualifications.

Physicians

All physicians have a doctoral degree in medicine and are licensed by the state medical board. Most physicians specialize in an area of medicine during their residency. Although any physician may refer a client to occupational therapy, some specialties are more common. Neurologists specialize in disorders of the nervous system. Orthopedists specialize in disorders of bones, joints, and ligaments. Physiatrists specialize in physical medicine and rehabilitation. Pediatricians specialize in treating children. Geriatricians specialize in treating older people. Cardiologists specialize in treating heart conditions. Psychiatrists specialize in treating mental health disorders. Some physicians are very knowledgeable about occupational therapy and its services, but others have minimal knowledge. There is no standard requirement in medical education regarding coverage of rehabilitation services in general or occupational therapy specifically. Occupational therapy practitioners need to ensure that physicians referring clients for occupational therapy services are knowledgeable about the services provided by occupational therapy in a given facility or program and are able to complete the required referral instructions.

Nurses

A registered nurse has a bachelor's degree or higher and is licensed by the state nursing board. Nurses are educated as generalists, but most become specialists in practice. Nurses may be able to refer a client to occupational therapy depending on the state licensing requirements. Whether they are the referral source or not, nurses in hospital settings are the most knowledgeable about the client's current status because they see the client throughout the day. Nurses often act as case managers to organize and monitor the care and treatment an individual client receives. Progress and problems are reported to the nurse case manager, who then coordinates any changes needed in the client's plan of care. Nurses who specialize in rehabilitation nursing are familiar with occupational therapy services, but nurses specializing in other services, such as neurology, orthopedics, pediatrics, gerontology, or cardiology, may have less knowledge of the role of occupational therapy with their clients. Nurses organize and coordinate the daily schedule for clients. They also see a client's needs and problems directly. Occupational therapy practitioners work closely with nurses to determine the best schedule for services and to assist in identifying the specific needs and problems of a particular client.

Nursing Assistants

Nursing assistants (e.g., licensed vocational nurses and licensed practical nurses) usually train at a community or junior college, and most states require them to be licensed. Their role is working with the registered nurses to carry out the client's plan of care. Nursing assistants often perform more of the "hands-on" client care, including getting the client ready to be seen by occupational therapy practitioners.

Nurse's Aides

Aides are trained on-the-job. They do the activities that do not require specialized training, such as bathing clients, setting up meal trays, and changing bed linens. They often interact more with the clients because they are in the client's room more of the time. A nurse's aide can provide useful information on a client's progress or lack of progress on a daily basis.

Physical Therapists

Physical therapists graduating today have a doctoral degree in physical therapy, but some physical therapy practitioners completed their education before the doctoral degree was required and thus have a master's degree. All are licensed by the state in which they practice. While many physical therapists work in hospitals or clinics, many also work in private practice and own an independent business specializing only in physical therapy, or specializing in rehabilitation services including occupational therapy and speech.

Dieticians and Nutritionists

Dieticians and nutritionists vary in their educational backgrounds depending on the state requirements. Some are licensed, and some are not. Their role is to plan and monitor meals that provide nutrition for clients, regardless of whether the client can eat normally or is being tube-fed. Occupational therapy practitioners often work with dieticians when clients have feeding disorders or need to learn to manage food preparation and eating habits related to a disorder, such as diabetes.

Psychologists

Psychologists usually have a doctoral degree in psychology and are licensed by the state board for psychology. Psychology includes many specialties but, in the hospital setting, the most common specialty is clinical psychology. The clinical psychologist's role is to monitor or evaluate client behavior and to suggest approaches to address client needs or facilitate better cooperation between the client and health care personnel. In schools, psychologists evaluate students' academic progress and learning styles. The results determine in what grade the student will be placed or which specialized educational program is best suited to the student's needs. Occupational therapy practitioners work with psychologists to develop a plan to modify behavior or to coordinate a program to improve student learning outcomes in the classroom.

Speech-Language Pathologists (Speech Therapists)

Speech therapists may have a bachelor's degree, but speech-language pathologists have a master's degree and certificate of clinical competency credentials. Speech-language pathologists are state licensed, but speech therapists may not be. The role of the speech therapist is to diagnosis and treat clients with voice, speech, and language disorders. Speech specialists may or may not be familiar with occupational therapy services, depending on where they received their education and their previous work experience. Occupational therapy practitioners may work with speech therapists in the school setting to improve communication skills using augmentative communication devices which are used with students with limited or no verbal speech.

Orthotists and Prosthetists

Credentialing for orthotists and prosthetists varies. Some are certified and licensed, but others are not, depending on the state requirements. Orthotists and prosthetists make orthopedic devices, including splints and braces. While occupational therapists make splints, the devices are usually designed for temporary wear and created from a special type of plastic. For the client who needs a permanent splint, one made of metal is a better choice, and the orthotist or prosthetist has the equipment to make splints. Orthotists and prosthetists spend much of their time making artificial limbs to replace amputated legs and arms. Orthotists and prosthetists may or may not be familiar with occupational therapy services, depending on where they received their training and their experience in working with rehabilitation programs. Occupational therapy practitioners work with orthotists and prosthetists to determine when temporary or permanent splints and braces best fulfill the needs of a client to provide stability or dynamic movement.

Special Education Teachers

Teachers of special education have at least a bachelor's degree, and many have a master's degree. They must also have a teaching certificate issued by the state in which they are employed. Special education teachers take courses related to teaching children with special needs, such as cerebral palsy or autism. Most special education teachers have learned about occupational therapy but may have a limited understanding of the role and relationship to classroom instruction. Occupational therapists consult with special education teachers to advise on how to help the student best perform in the educational environment, including modification of behavior and adaptation of the learning environment.

General Education Teachers

All teachers have at least a bachelor's degree, although many have a master's degree. In addition, they must have a teaching certificate issued by the state in which they teach. Teachers who majored in regular education rarely learn about occupational therapy services. They need to be informed about the cooperative and consultative role occupational therapy practitioners provide to modify behavior and facilitate better learning environments, including computer-assisted instruction for children with special needs who are otherwise able to function in the regular classroom.

School Principals and Administrators

Most principals and administrators have been regular education teachers before becoming principals or administrators. They become familiar with the rules and regulations concerning special education and about children with special needs, but often require additional information to understand the role of occupational therapy in the school system and how occupational therapy practitioners can assist teachers to modify behavior and adapt the learning environment to better suit the abilities of students with special needs.

Social Workers

Social workers usually have a master's degree or higher and are licensed by the state. Most work-for-state offices are responsible for child care and welfare, or are responsible for coordinating the discharge from a hospital to another setting, such as a nursing home. Social workers typically do not learn about occupational therapy services unless they have specialized training in hospital or health care services, such as mental health. Occupational therapy practitioners may coordinate with social workers to assess housing appropriate for persons with disabilities or co-lead a group of people with substance disorders to improve the clients' ability to function in the community.

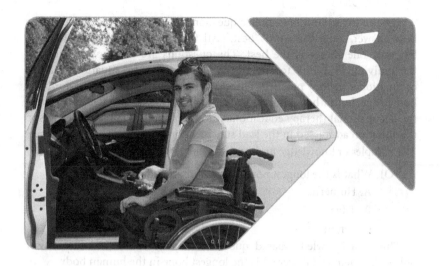

5

Becoming an Occupational Therapist

TAKING THE CERTIFICATION EXAM

All states require individuals who want to become licensed as occupational therapists or occupational therapy assistants to take the examination administered by the National Board for Certification in Occupational Therapy (NBCOT). The examination is given online at testing centers, and the individual must have an NBCOT code, which is provided after the NBCOT has verified the individual's educational qualifications. The occupational therapist examination is composed mostly of multiple-choice questions and a few clinical simulation items. The occupational therapy assistant examination is composed only of multiple-choice questions. The multiple-choice questions each have a lead statement or question followed by three or four choices, of which one is correct. A few questions on the occupational therapy assistant examination have a six-choice option with multiple correct answers.

Stein, F., & Reed, K. L.
Occupational Therapy: A Guide for Prospective
Students, Consumers, and Advocates (pp. 57-61).
© 2021 Taylor & Francis Group.

For the three- and four-choice questions, only one of the choices is the **best** answer. Note the word "best." All the choices may seem plausible, but only one choice is the **best**. The questions are designed to measure the individual's ability to apply knowledge to specific situations seen in occupational therapy practice. Therefore, the questions do not ask for basic knowledge, but rather assume the examinee knows certain facts learned in the occupational therapy educational program and can apply those facts to the situation addressed in the lead statement or question.

Examples of knowledge and applied questions are given here.

Q1. What is the longest bone in the human body?

    A. Humerus

    B. Tibia

    C. Femur

This is a knowledge-based question. Anyone could find the answer online. The femur (answer C) is the longest bone in the human body.

Q2. Mrs. James has fractured her femur, or hip bone. The occupational therapy practitioner may recommend she use which of the following adaptive devices while her hip heals?

    A. Enlarged spoon handle

    B. Sock aid

    C. Button hook

This is an applied question requiring that information be acquired and applied to a specific situation. Note that all the answers are names of adaptive devices that Mrs. James might use. However, the occupational therapy practitioner knows that a client with a hip fracture will be instructed to limit the amount of bending at the hip while the fracture heals. Putting on socks requires bending over or down to place the sock over the toes and foot. A sock aid allows the sock to be pulled over a frame that has long handles attached so that the sock can be placed on the foot without bending the body at the hip. Therefore, the best answer is sock aid (answer B).

Q3. The adult human body is composed of how many bones?

    A. 206

    B. 182

    C. 345

    D. 97

This question is another knowledge-based question. The answer can be found online. The correct answer is 206 (answer A).

Q4. Mrs. Lee recently broke her radius during a fall. The occupational therapy practitioner should evaluate her ability to move which joint while performing daily activities?

A. Knee

B. Shoulder

C. Elbow

D. Wrist

Movement occurs in all of these joints, so all are possible answers, but which is the best answer? The occupational therapy practitioner knows that the radius is one of bones that forms the wrist joint, and that when a fracture site is immobilized in a cast during the healing process, that joint often becomes stiff and does not move easily during the performance of daily activities. The practitioner therefore needs to evaluate how well the wrist joint (answer D) is moving following the healing of the radius, and may recommend activities designed to increase the joint's mobility.

Q5. The letters ADHD stand for:

A. Action deficiency and height deficit

B. Attention deficit hyperactivity disorder

C. Activity dysfunction hypothyroid disease

D. Arousal difficulty hyporesponsive dysfunction

This is another knowledge-based question. The correct answer is attention deficit hyperactivity disorder (answer B).

Q6. Jason has ADHD. His teacher consults with the school-based occupational therapy practitioner because Jason is not completing his in-class seatwork on time. Which of the following environmental modifications might help Jason better manage his symptoms of ADHD and attend to this seatwork? Select "Yes" next to those options that are appropriate. Select "No" if the option is not appropriate. Either "Yes" or "No" must be selected for every option.

Yes	No	
☐	☐	Enlarge the size of the print on the worksheets
☐	☐	Place the table or desk facing a wall
☐	☐	Have the teacher's aide assist him
☐	☐	Use noise-cancelling headphones
☐	☐	Make the lessons easier to complete
☐	☐	Use as much natural light as possible

This question is designed as a clinical simulation. The clinical reasoning process is to decrease the amount of sensory stimulation in Jason's environment. Reducing the contact with others by placing the desk against a wall, wearing noise-cancelling headphones, and using natural light as opposed to florescent light are all methods of reducing sensory stimulation. Enlarging the size of the print on the worksheets is not needed because Jason does not have a visual deficit. A teacher's aide is not needed because Jason is not physically handicapped and does not have a learning disability. Making the lessons easier is not necessary because Jason has normal intelligence.

Adapted from the NBCOT *Certification Exam Handbook 2020*.

So what kind of information should an occupational therapy student study to prepare for the exam? Students often assume they should cram as many facts as possible into their heads. As the sample questions should suggest, facts are of limited help. More important is the ability to apply the facts to problems seen by occupational therapy practitioners in clinic, home, or community situations. Thinking in terms of case studies may be more helpful. Given a set of facts:

- What actions would an occupational therapy practitioner take to provide occupational therapy services to an individual, a group, or a community?
- What would be the best evaluation or assessment procedure to assess the problem or problems?
- How should data be analyzed and interpreted?
- What goal or goals should be set in the intervention plan?
- What intervention methods or devices would be best to use?
- How would the client's progress be measured?
- What regulations, standards of practice, or responsibilities should be followed?
- How should practitioners collaborate with other professionals and colleagues?

All these questions require the application of information to determine the best answer. Note the focus on solving problems: What information should be gathered and analyzed? What evaluation procedures should be used? What goals should be set? What methods or devices should be used? What will measure the progress? What regulations or standards must be observed in working with clients, colleagues, and administrators? Facts can provide the answer to a knowledge-based question, but the ability to use information to solve a problem provides the answer to an application question.

More information about preparing and taking the certification examination is available in the NBCOT *Certification Exam Handbook,* available online at www.nbcot.org. The categories of questions for both the occupational therapist and occupational therapy assistant are listed and described along with the percentage or proportion of test items devoted to that category. For both examinations, the largest percentage or proportion of test items is developed to focus on intervention, including selection, implementation, and management of the intervention process. Evaluation and gathering information form the second-largest category.

The exact number of questions on the examinations is not provided because the number changes from time to time. Refer to the NBCOT *Certification Exam Handbook* for the exact number of questions. The handbook is revised each year to provide the most up-to-date information regarding the rules and regulations for taking the examination.

An astute reader may have guessed that completing the certification examination requires a brain that can think clearly and concisely, as opposed to one that is crammed with facts. Deprivation of sleep and food is not recommended. The night before taking the examination should be devoted to getting some quality sleep, not last-minute studying. Eating a good meal and getting some exercise can help the process of getting ready before reporting to the test center.

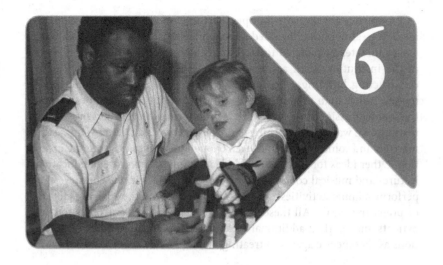

What Is the History of Occupational Therapy?

OCCUPATIONS AS A THERAPEUTIC AGENT

Occupational therapy as a profession had its beginning as an alternative to the prevailing ideas and methods of treating people with mental and behavioral disorders. In the 18th and 19th centuries, prevailing ideas regarding the etiology of mental illness were speculative. They included misplaced notions, such as that people with mental or behavioral problems had been put under a spell, had been poisoned by some unknown force, were possessed by demons, or were being punished for sins by a deity. A common belief was that people with mental illness were incurable and should be removed permanently from society for the benefit of both the individual and the community. Methods of treatment might include being put in isolation or imprisoned, chained to a wall to prevent escape, beaten to get rid of the spell or demons, given laxatives to get rid of the poisons, or any combination thereof.

Stein, F., & Reed, K. L.
Occupational Therapy: A Guide for Prospective Students, Consumers, and Advocates (pp. 63-70).
© 2021 Taylor & Francis Group.

Progressive thinkers in Europe and the United States tried alternative ideas of treatment that included a humanitarian approach. One idea was to assign inmates or patients to work tasks associated with the maintenance of the institution, such as mowing the lawn, working in agriculture, or constructing buildings. The rationale was often more economic to save money, rather than therapeutic to aid recovery, but some doctors observed that patients assigned to such work tasks improved faster than those left on institutional wards with nothing to do. Patients who got better were easier to manage, and some were deemed well enough to be released from the institution. Other ideas for treatment included having patients attend educational lectures and musical concerts, go for walks and rides in the countryside, or perform manual activities, such as sweeping, cleaning, repairing clothing, or preparing meals. All these occupations had positive outcomes for some patients and sparked additional ideas about the potential value of occupations as therapeutic agents in treating mental and behavioral disorders.

OCCUPATIONS AS THERAPY

Beginning in 1905, Herbert James Hall, MD, in Marblehead, Massachusetts, began writing about using handcrafts as treatment for mental conditions. In 1910, he published the first research article on the effectiveness of such treatment in the *Journal of the American Medical Association*.

In 1906, Susan Edith Tracy, a nurse, started training nurses to use handcrafts with patients at the Adams Nervine Hospital in Jamaica Plain, Massachusetts. In 1910, she published *Invalid Occupations*, the first textbook on using occupations as treatment.

Julia Lathrop had been a member of the Illinois State Board of Control and observed the idleness of patients in state institutions. In 1908, she started a course for nurses and attendants. The course was designed to provide training in the use of handcrafts, games, music, and exercises so that patients' time was filled in more constructive activities and occupations.

In 1911, William Rush Dunton, Jr., MD, began training nurses to use occupations with patients at the Sheppard and Enoch Pratt Hospital in Baltimore, Maryland.

In 1915, the Illinois Society for Mental Hygiene in Chicago, Illinois, opened an outpatient clinic called the Occupation Center. The director, Eleanor Clarke Slagle, a student of Julia Lathrop's, stated that people with disorders, including physical, mental, tubercular, and cardiac conditions, were accepted for training or retraining to be able to earn a living. Special attention was made to observe and train the clients in occupations that were of interest and fitted their individual talents and abilities.

In the same year, George Edward Barton, an architect with tuberculosis living in Clifton Springs, New York, published an article suggesting the term *occupational therapy* be used to describe the use of occupations in a manner designed to parallel the use of the term *drug therapy*. In other words, Barton suggested there should be an occupation that provided a therapeutic effect equal to or similar to each drug currently being used to treat patients. While his theory may have been flawed, his term remains. Although many names had been used previously to encompass the idea of using occupation as a therapeutic agent, Barton's term *occupational therapy* rapidly gained acceptance and remains the name of the profession today.

STARTING A PROFESSION

In 1917, six people agreed to meet in Clifton Springs to discuss creating an organization devoted to studying the use of occupations as therapeutic agents and promoting occupational therapy as a profession. Barton, who had coined the term occupational therapy, hosted the meeting. Susan Cox Johnson worked on Blackwell Island with immigrants whom immigration authorities considered to have mental disorders. Thomas Bessell Kidner, an architect and manual arts teacher, was from Canada and had experience with setting up retraining programs for injured soldiers returning from the war in Europe. Isabel Newton was Barton's secretary. Dr. Dunton, who trained nurses in Maryland, and Slagle, director of the Illinois Society for Mental Hygiene, also attended. Published authors Dr. Hall and Tracy did not attend the founding meeting but were active as the resulting association progressed.

At the founding meeting, the new organization was named the National Society for the Promotion of Occupational Therapy and in 1921 was renamed the American Occupational Therapy Association (AOTA). A national office was established in 1922 in New York City and quickly became a hub for activities related to occupational therapy. For many years, the operational definition of occupational therapy was the one provided by H. A. Pattison, MD, as "any activity, mental or physical, definitely prescribed for the distinct purpose of contributing to and hastening recovery from disease or injury."

WORLD WAR I

In early 1918, the U.S. Army developed what were called *reconstruction services* to treat injured soldiers. The term for the people doing the treating was *reconstruction aide* (RA). RAs were civilians who volunteered to serve their country by providing reconstructive services that today would be called occupational therapists, physical therapists, social workers, and librarians. Nurses were called nurses, but the other professions were simply grouped together under the name RA. The RAs served in Europe, especially in France, and in the reconstruction camps set up in the United States following the end of the war. The use of RAs trained in occupational therapy was recognized as an effective treatment modality in the military hospitals. As former military physicians began to transition out of the military, they promoted the use of occupational therapy in civilian hospitals, veterans facilities, and state institutions, which increased the need for trained occupational therapy personnel.

DEVELOPMENT OF EDUCATIONAL AND REGULATORY STANDARDS

Educational standards for the training of occupational therapists were first adopted by the AOTA in 1923 and published in the official journal, *Archives of Occupational Therapy,* in 1924. The standards established the basic pattern for the curriculum, which included medical lectures, arts and crafts courses to learn the application of occupation to disorders, and practice training to learn to work directly with clients. In 1935, the AOTA began developing educational standards in cooperation with the American Medical Association. Initially, in 1938, five occupational therapy programs were accredited. Regulatory standards to establish the qualifications for practitioners began with registration in 1932. Initially, some practitioners were registered based on their practice experience, but after 1939, all practitioners were required to have completed an accredited educational course in occupational therapy. Later, practitioners were also required to take and pass an examination first mandated in 1946.

WORLD WAR II

When the United States entered the second World War in December 1941, the profession of occupational therapy was inadequately prepared to meet the needs of injured servicemen and servicewomen. The Great Depression had reduced or eliminated the number of occupational therapy positions in many hospitals and institutions. Membership in the AOTA was 1,207 in 1940, but only eight therapists worked in military hospitals. There were six accredited educational programs, and one of those was in Canada; by 1945, there were 16 accredited programs. To meet the need short-term, war emergency courses were established for people who already had a college degree but lacked training in applying occupation as a therapeutic agent and knowledge of conditions seen frequently in occupational therapy clinics. An outgrowth of the war was the need to recognize specialized practice. The practice training required of student occupational therapists was expanded to include orthopedics, pediatrics, tuberculosis, general medicine, and surgery, as well as mental disorders.

POST-WAR EXPANSION AND GROWTH

Following the end of World War II, there was an increased interest in physical rehabilitation, which had been successful in military hospitals and was then expanded to civilian and community programs. Occupational therapy practice expanded to include diseases of the nervous system, such as brain injuries, stroke, and peripheral injuries affecting the hand. In 1952, the World Federation of Occupational Therapists was formed. The United States was one of 10 founding countries. As the recognition of occupational therapy increased, the need for an additional level of personnel was recognized to work beside occupational therapists. The occupational therapy assistant role was formally established in 1958.

CHANGING WITH THE TIMES

The passage of federal legislation, including the Community Mental Health and Mental Retardation Act (1963), Medicare (1965), Medicaid (1966), and the Allied Health Act (1966), had a profound effect on the practice of occupational therapy. As practice in mental health moved from institutions to communities, and drug therapy replaced the emphasis on developing and maintaining habits and routines, occupational therapy positions in mental health facilities decreased. At the same time, the availability of insurance coverage for medical conditions requiring physical rehabilitation services further expanded the practice in occupational therapy in the area of physical disorders. More nursing homes offered occupational therapy services, and more home services were available. The Allied Health Act provided funds to start additional occupational therapy educational programs, which accelerated the expansion of available programs to educate both occupational therapists and assistants. Drug therapy also changed the delivery of services for people with tuberculosis from the sanatorium to the community, although no federal legislation was involved. In the early 1960s, the requirement was dropped for students to have practice training in facilities treating tuberculosis. The development of the polio vaccine in the 1950s changed the delivery of services to children with acute poliomyelitis to providing services to adults with post-polio conditions.

The 1960s also included changes in the practice theory and methods. The theory called *habit training* had been used in mental hospitals since Slagle had initiated it into the New York State hospitals in 1922. As other practice areas developed and different ideas about treatment evolved, new theories emerged. Occupational behavior as a general theory of practice was advanced, as were the beginning ideas of sensory integration.

FEDERAL AND STATE INFLUENCES

The passage of the Education for All Handicapped Children Act (1975) rapidly introduced occupational therapy services into public and private school settings to help children with disabilities participate more fully in their education. Thus, another change in practice settings occurred as occupational therapy expanded from hospitals and institutions, to nursing homes, and to school settings.

As occupational therapy services were introduced into more legislation, the issue of state licensure also increased, because licensure was often the criterion for inclusion or exclusion in the legislation. The growing influence of federal legislation prompted the AOTA to move its headquarters from New York City to the Washington, DC, area in 1972. In 1974, the AOTA started preparing a model practice act to guide states and jurisdictions in writing licensure legislation. Puerto Rico was the first jurisdiction to adopt a license law, and Florida and New York would become the first states to pass laws requiring all occupational therapists to be state-licensed, but initially the laws did not include occupational therapy assistants. Along with state licensure was the growing awareness that a professional code of ethics was needed. The AOTA adopted the first code of ethics in 1977.

CHANGING PRACTICE TRENDS

Although occupational therapy had started practice with handcrafts, games, dance, music, and physical exercises, by the 1980s all these modalities had largely been replaced. Occupational therapy now focused on remediating the effects of disorders and disabilities using methods such as activities of daily living and self-care activities developed in the 1950s, homemaking skills, work safety and injury prevention techniques, role performance skills, prevocational training, therapeutic exercises, neurodevelopmental techniques, and physical agent modalities. However, the concept of purposeful and meaningful occupation remained a core belief. Therapeutic exercises, neurodevelopmental techniques, and physical agent modalities were considered preparatory activities designed to prepare the client to better perform the occupations needed to participate successfully in everyday life to the greatest extent possible.

Federal legislation continued to influence practice. In 1980, Medicare was expanded to cover outpatient rehabilitation services including occupational therapy, and hospice care was covered in 1982. Legal cases related to antitrust issues began to challenge the status of professional organizations, such as the AOTA, that regulated both accreditation of educational programs and registration or certification of practitioners. As a result, the AOTA decided to maintain the accreditation process in-house, but create a separate organization for certification. Created in 1986, the American Occupational Therapy Certification Board became the National Board for Certification in Occupational Therapy in 1996.

EDUCATIONAL STANDARDS AND PRACTICE REVISED

In 1994, the accreditation process changed again as the AOTA formally separated from the cooperative agreement with the American Medical Association that had started in 1933, and created the Accreditation Council for Occupational Therapy Education. The Accreditation Council for Occupational Therapy Education became responsible for accrediting both professional and technically educated occupational therapy practitioners, and new educational standards were adopted for both the occupational therapist and occupational therapy assistant. These standards would be updated again in 1999 when the AOTA changed the entry educational requirement from a bachelor's degree to a master's degree; this took effect in 2007. By 1999, 40 states plus the District of Columbia and Puerto Rico had professional-level education programs, and 48 had technical education programs. Only Alaska had neither. Between 1938 and 1999, the accredited educational programs in occupational therapy had expanded from four states to 40.

A membership survey in 1990 showed that the most common problems treated by occupational therapy personnel were stroke/hemiplegia, developmental delay, cerebral palsy, hand injury, and learning disability. Self-employed practitioners or those in private practice were increasing. The highest ratio of therapists to population could be found in Colorado, Massachusetts, New Hampshire, North Dakota, and Wisconsin. The lowest ratios were in the southwestern and southern states.

CENTENNIAL VISION

In 2003, members of the AOTA began to look ahead to 2017, the 100th anniversary of the founding of the AOTA, by creating a vision statement that read: "We envision that occupational therapy is a powerful, widely recognized, science-driven, and evidence-based profession with a globally connected and diverse workforce meeting society's occupational needs." The vision statement was accompanied by the adoption of a branding statement designed to identify the profession. The statement, adopted in 2008, reads: "Occupational Therapy: Living Life to Its Fullest." The AOTA also developed the *Occupational Therapy Practice Framework* to "affirm and articulate the focus of occupational therapy on occupation and daily life activities and the application of an intervention process that facilitates engagement in occupation to support participation." The *Framework* is updated about every 5 years to ensure it encompasses and reflects current occupational therapy practice.

INTO THE SECOND CENTURY

Occupational therapy practitioners celebrated the 100th anniversary of the founding in 2017 at the annual meeting in Philadelphia, Pennsylvania. Just 2 years before, the requirement for a professional licensure was achieved in all 50 states and three jurisdictions (District of Columbia, Guam, and Puerto Rico) for both occupational therapists and assistants. In addition, the AOTA adopted a statement designed to outline the distinct value of occupational therapy services: "Occupational therapy's distinct value is to improve health and quality of life though facilitating participation and engagement in occupations, the meaningful, necessary, and familiar activities of everyday life. Occupational therapy is client-centered, achieves positive outcomes, and is cost-effective."

Thus the profession of occupational therapy continues to define itself in society and culture in terms of its roles and functions in the delivery of health care, prevention, rehabilitation, and health education services. Although the profession once relied primarily on medicine and physicians, it has developed its own standards and scope of practice as an independent profession that cooperates not only with physicians but also with other professionals, such as educators, psychologists, physical therapists, speech pathologists, and social workers, to provide services designed to help people live better lives and participate more fully in their community.

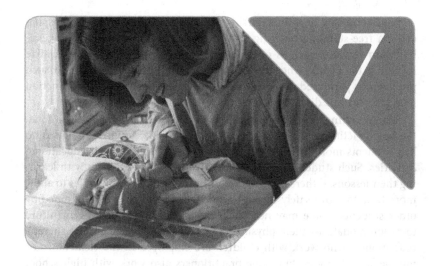

Where Do Occupational Therapists Work?

Occupational therapists and assistants work in many different settings depending on the needs and goals of the people being served. The three primary work settings are hospitals, long-term care or skilled nursing facilities, and schools. Collectively these three settings account for about two-thirds of the work settings that employ occupational therapy personnel.

The hospitals may have specialized units, such as acute care for adults, neonatal intensive care for infants, pediatric, hospice care, inpatient rehabilitation, or outpatient rehabilitation. Specialized units provide services tailored to one specific type of need. For example, neonatal intensive care units specialize in providing care for infants born prematurely or those with disorders that cause difficulty with breathing, feeding, and normal development.

Stein, F., & Reed, K. L.
Occupational Therapy: A Guide for Prospective
Students, Consumers, and Advocates (pp. 71-74).
© 2021 Taylor & Francis Group.

Long-term care or skilled nursing facilities may be attached to a hospital or be a free-standing building that provides medical, nursing, and rehabilitation services, such as occupational therapy. Such facilities specialize in caring for people who are unable to care for themselves due to such problems as paralyzed muscles, loss of memory, or general loss of function related to chronic disease.

School settings include public and private institutions. Occupational therapy practitioners working in schools provide services designed to help students more fully benefit from and participate in their educational activities. Such students may need assistive technology to help with learning their lessons. Others may need modifications to their schedules to allow more time to move safely through the building without being bumped by other students. Some may need help modifying and arranging furniture to accommodate to their physical condition. Most occupational therapy practitioners who work with children are employed in the elementary or middle school grades, but some practitioners also work with high school transitional programs designed to help students with disabilities move from school to work settings and from home to community living.

Other work settings include freestanding outpatient facilities, home health services, early intervention programs, mental health and behavioral disorder facilities, and academic settings. Freestanding outpatient facilities most often provide rehabilitation services that combine occupational therapy, physical therapy, and speech-language pathology. Other services, such as audiology, recreation, music, art, or drama, may be available. Freestanding rehabilitation facilities may provide services for people who have been released from a hospital setting, or for people whose needs do not require hospitalization but do require specialized treatment.

Home health, as the term implies, is a service delivered in the home where the person lives. Such service is not only tailored to the person's needs and goals, but can also be tried out and practiced in the actual environment where the person lives and performs many of the activities of daily living. Hospital settings rarely, if ever, can duplicate the home living environment. For many people, home services determine whether they can function in the home or will require the specialized care of a skilled nursing home.

Early intervention programs may be provided in freestanding facilities or be housed in a community service center or a school building. Such programs are designed for toddlers and preschoolers who are at-risk for developmental delays, typically ages 3 to 5 years, to improve skills related to daily living activities and to prepare them to participate in the school environment.

Mental health facilities may be located in a freestanding building, within a unit in a general hospital, in a specialized community-based program, or as part of a multiservice community service program. Such mental health programs may provide general services for many types of mental and behavior disorders or may specialize in treating only one type of problem, such as depression, alcoholism, or opioid addiction.

Occupational therapy personnel who work in academic settings may be located in educational institutions, such as universities, colleges, or technical training facilities. Their job is teaching students, at the professional and technical level, the knowledge, skills, and attitudes needed to become occupational therapy practitioners. Some academics work full-time at the educational institution, but many teach part-time, while also working in another setting.

Finally there are highly specialized work settings, such as driving rehabilitation programs, home modification programs, industrial rehabilitation or work programs, prison or forensic programs, research centers, sheltered workshops, and supported employment. Practitioners who work in such programs may be employed full-time or part-time. Driving rehabilitation programs are designed to assess and train or retrain people who want to get a driver's license for the first time or keep the one they have. Some may have lost function due to illness, such as stroke or head injury. Teenagers with developmental disorders may need special assessment and training to determine if driving a vehicle is within their visual-motor coordination skills and cognitive judgment for safety issues.

Home modification programs are designed to assess and make recommendations for altering a home and its surroundings to better accommodate a person's ability to function safely and effectively. While physical barriers, such as door openings that are too narrow to permit a wheelchair to pass through or stairs that cannot be climbed safely, are common, other problems, such as inadequate lighting and doorbells that cannot be heard, also exist. Usually, practitioners specializing in home modification work with architects or builders to determine whether structural changes to a home meet legal codes or what materials will provide strength, safety, and endurance.

Industrial rehabilitation or work programs are designed to provide opportunities for people to try out work activities under the supervision of practitioners trained to promote safety and prevent additional injury or dysfunction. People participating in such programs may have been injured on the job or had an illness, such as a stroke, heart attack, or cancer, that changed their physical or mental abilities. The program includes typical work situations, such as lifting, reaching, climbing, walking with objects in one's arms, and placing such objects on the correct shelf or in the right box. The amount of time a person can work, the weight of materials to be handled, and the ability to replicate the task safely and accurately must all be evaluated.

Working in prisons or forensic settings requires the practitioner to become familiar with the rules and regulations of these facilities as well as to provide services designed to increase skills in conforming to community standards of behavior and cultural norms. For the occupational therapy practitioner, the prisoner's actual crime is not usually the issue. Rather, the issues are the underlying physical, mental, or social interaction problems that contribute to a situation in which community rules and regulations are broken, and whether the person can master the skills and adjust behavior to function in the community again.

Research centers are most often located in colleges or universities, but may be located in an industry such as one that manufactures rehabilitation equipment. Occupational therapy personnel working in a research center usually have specialized advanced training in a specific area of practice. In addition, the research-focused occupational therapist must learn the rules and regulations regarding people participating as research subjects to avoid injury or harm during their participation in the research study. Development of skills in writing grants to secure funds for the research projects may also be required.

Sheltered workshops offer work opportunities for people who cannot meet the demands of regular employment. Such people may not be able to work rapidly or accurately enough, or may not be able to carry out the number of instructions required to complete a task. Sheltered workshops provide tasks that can be adjusted to meet the abilities of the workers, as opposed to requiring the worker to meet the requirements of the job. Supported employment settings include on-site supervisors who can oversee the worker's performance at all times and provide immediate guidance or correction as needed. Such on-site supervision allows a person who has had a change in health status to return to work in settings where the employer might be otherwise cautious about allowing the person to return. Alternatively, such on-site supervision may allow a person to try out for a job where the employer might otherwise refuse to allow the person to be employed.

The work settings described here are typical but not inclusive. Occupational therapy education in the knowledge of human occupation and skills in occupational performance provides a broad base in solving problems people may encounter and need assistance performing. Therefore, the job market is often in a state of flux. Over the years, many job opportunities have come and gone. However, history has also demonstrated that if one area of practice closes, another—or two or three—will open.

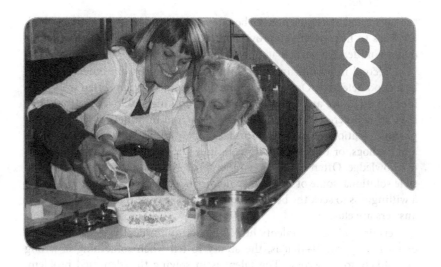

Personal Characteristics of Occupational Therapists

INTERESTS, ABILITIES, TALENTS, AND SKILLS

Certain interests, abilities, talents, or skills increase the potential for enjoying and succeeding in performing the work tasks associated with a particular profession. Occupational therapy is no different.

First and foremost, occupational therapists and assistants work directly with people. An interest in people is critical, as is the ability to interact in social situations. Also important is the ability to adjust to changes in social interaction situations. People who are ill or who are struggling to meet the challenges of everyday living are not always happy, in a good mood, or in a pleasant frame of mind. Occupational therapists and assistants must be able to adjust their interactions to acknowledge the mood of their clients while at the same time supporting and encouraging participation that will address the goals to be achieved through occupational therapy. Occupational

Stein, F., & Reed, K. L.
Occupational Therapy: A Guide for Prospective Students, Consumers, and Advocates (pp. 75-80).
© 2021 Taylor & Francis Group.

therapists and assistants need to be interested in and have the ability to look for ways to help people improve their health and wellness, promote their quality of life, and participate more fully in everyday life.

A second important interest is that of investigator—in other words, to be a good detective. Occupational therapists and assistants often work with ideas that require an extensive amount of thinking and investigating. They have to be interested in searching for facts and information to figure out possible solutions. Facts and information may be available online, in books and catalogs, or by talking with colleagues or experts in a particular field of knowledge. Often occupational therapists and assistants have to try possible solutions, some of which may not be successful. Investigation includes a willingness to seek the best answers but also tolerate that sometimes good answers are elusive.

Certain abilities or talents help. The ability to identify that a problem exists is important—that is, the ability to tell when something is wrong or is likely to go wrong. The talent is in solving the identified problem. Occupational therapists and assistants often spend time figuring out how to modify a task to permit a person to perform it when the typical or expected way simply does not work. Solving the problem may require analyzing how a person can change an approach to the task, how the task might be modified or simplified, or how the environment (e.g., furniture or lighting) might be rearranged or enhanced. People who enjoy identifying a problem and the challenge of working on a solution may enjoy becoming occupational therapists or assistants.

Another important ability is concerned with reasoning. *Deductive reasoning* is the ability to apply general rules to specific problems to produce answers that make sense. *Inductive reasoning* is the ability to combine pieces of information to form general rules or conclusions. For example, if a person keeps dropping their fork while eating dinner, deductive reasoning suggests that larger handles are easier to hold onto than the typical flat, thin, and thus small handles of forks. Inductive reasoning looks for ways to increase the size of the fork handle. What if a wash rag were wrapped around the handle to make it large? What if forks with larger handles could be ordered online? Would either or both solutions improve the ability of the person to grasp and hold on to the fork while eating? Are other solutions possible? The ability to reason both deductively and inductively contributes to the ability to identify a problem and create a solution.

A third ability is oral comprehension and oral expression. *Oral comprehension* is the ability to listen and understand information and ideas presented through spoken words and sentences. *Oral expression* is the ability to communicate information and ideas in speaking so others will understand. Both are important to occupational therapists and assistants. For example, a nursing supervisor might say, "Mrs. Bradley dropped her fork three times during dinner last night. I don't know what is happening." Listening to the nurse should suggest to the occupational therapist or assistant that there is a problem that the nurse would like addressed. After observing the problem and identifying solutions, the occupational therapist or assistant might speak with the nurse suggesting that several solutions may be tried and asking if Mrs. Bradley can be approached to try out one or more of the suggested options.

A fourth ability is teaching, educating, and instructing. Although occupational therapists and assistants do not need a teaching certificate to practice occupational therapy, during the performance of their job duties, they do a lot of teaching, educating, and instructing. People with disabilities need to learn skills and perform tasks that a typically developing or nondisabled person does not need to learn or has learned many years ago. Parents, family members, and other caregivers need to learn how to care for people with disabilities. Occupational therapists and assistants, along with other rehabilitation personnel, become a primary source of such education. Teaching requires dividing or breaking down the occupation or activity into tasks or units that can be taught and repeated until the learner has mastered the tasks and can put them together to perform the occupation in total. Teaching requires motivating the learner to learn and having the patience to repeat the instruction and watch the learner practice until the task is mastered. Teaching may also require revising the teaching strategy if the first approach does not result in the client learning as expected. Teaching strategies can include verbal or voice instruction, gestures such as pointing to an item, or demonstrations showing how the task is done. Often a combination of all three strategies is needed.

A fifth ability is writing. Most occupational therapists and assistants will not become award-winning, famous authors, but they will write the equivalent of hundreds of pages throughout their career. Writing skills are needed for documenting information, such as the results of an assessment, an intervention plan including goals and desired outcomes, the results of the intervention plans with progress toward goals and outcomes, revisions of intervention plans, discharge plans and summaries, instructions for caregivers to follow, and justifications to payers for reimbursement. Checklists often reduce the actual amount of words written, but some details cannot be reduced to checkmarks. Most documentation is performed on a computer, although some paperwork is inevitable. In general, the writing must be concise and to the point. Documentation is not a literary assignment to write the Great American Novel. Documentation should be factual, accurate, complete, and timely. More words are not necessarily better, but leaving important details out is not a winning formula either.

A sixth ability is mental flexibility, which involves being able to change thinking and doing strategies quickly, to move on with what needs to be done without too much fuss or muss. The best-laid plans often do not happen as planned. Occupational therapists and assistants learn to have alternative strategies available at all times. If plan A does not work, plan B will be tried, and maybe plans C or D. Sometimes the time schedule must be changed, sometimes clients come late for appointments, and sometimes clients are in a very bad mood and just say "no" even when asked nicely. Although the concepts of managing time, being organized, and planning ahead are good strategies, they may have to give way to unforeseen changes in the immediate situation.

KNOWLEDGE, SKILLS, AND ATTITUDES

Specialized knowledge and skills form the basis of most professions. Unlike other professions, for the occupational therapy professions, knowledge will include both biological and social sciences. Biological sciences include zoology (high school), anatomy, physiology, kinesiology, neuroanatomy, and neurophysiology (college). Social sciences include psychology, abnormal psychology, child development, learning and teaching, and sociology. Courses in health and wellness, pathology of disease and illness, and medical conditions and treatment will also be included. Therapy courses will focus on evaluation and intervention or rehabilitation of physical and behavioral dysfunction.

Skill courses will address the three aspects critical to the application of occupational therapy: the person (client), the occupation (activity), and the environment (human and nonhuman). The person or client may be an individual but may also be an organization, a business, or a government entity. The occupation or activity includes anything people do in their lives, including activities done with other people and with animals. The environment includes social interactions with others (human or animal) and the interface between humans and the built, manufactured, or natural environment.

The first focus is on how to assess the client's problems, needs, and goals. The second focus is on how to plan and implement an intervention program to effectively and efficiently address the problems, needs, goals, and desired outcomes. Finally, the third focus is on measuring if the outcomes have been achieved and planning any necessary follow-up.

Technology skills form an increasingly important part of the occupational therapist's or assistant's repertoire. Computer skills form a large part of the technology skill set. Word processing and spreadsheet use will be expected. Other computer skills include use of software for graphics, photo imaging, enlarging and changing fonts, internet browsing, medical condition monitoring, email, music or sound editing, optical character reading, voice recognition, web page creating and editing, and controlling (e.g., opening or closing, and starting or stopping) external devices and appliances.

Another technology involves the material to make splints. A splint is a device used to immobilize and align one or more joints *(static splint),* to assist in certain motions *(dynamic splint),* or to prevent deformity and loss of function. Splints may be used temporarily, periodically, or permanently. Although splints can be made from metal, most splints fashioned by occupational therapists are made from types of plastic, but may be covered with cloth materials to reduce friction with the client's skin. A typical splint made by an occupational therapist is designed for the hand, forearm, elbow, neck, or face, but, especially in children, other body parts may require splinting. Knowledge of how joints are normally aligned and move is critical to making splints, as is concern for care of skin to avoid damage. Skill is required to mold the splinting material to the joint or joints and provide fasteners to keep the splint in place.

A third technology is rehabilitation equipment, such as wheelchairs, scooters, walkers, or other mobility aids. To be of maximum benefit, the mobility aid must be fixed to the client's exact measurement as though it were a tailored garment. Such equipment is often expensive and must meet certain requirements to be covered by insurance. Knowledge of types of mobility aids, their availability, and their use is important. If the mobility aid is to provide maximum benefit, skill in measuring the person correctly and in recommending the best type is essential.

In addition, occupational therapists and assistants deal with a group of technologies known as adapted devices, which may include eating utensils, grooming and dressing aids, modified handle grips for tools, overhead pulley systems, and adapted equipment for work and leisure activities. These devices are designed to help perform everyday tasks required in daily life, work, or play. Occupational therapists and assistants help clients become aware of the availability, provide opportunities to try out devices, and provide training as needed. Knowledge of availability and use is important, as is the skill in teaching proper use, care, and safety precautions.

Attitudes are also important. Occupational therapists and assistants need to believe in and value each person for being an individual, regardless of physical, mental, or social attributes. No one is useless, incurable, a "basket case," or unworthy of attention, care, and hope. All individuals can learn and change their behavior, although some can learn and change more than others, and in some cases, the major change may be to the environmental conditions in which the person lives. In occupational therapy practice, there is no predetermined ceiling on what a person can do or accomplish. The job of occupational therapists and assistants is to make performance and achievement possible without putting arbitrary limits on either. Over the years, people with disabilities and developmental delays have been underestimated. Some have performed and achieved beyond what anyone thought possible. Occupational therapists and assistants believe in possibilities and try to figure out ways to make the possible a reality. Success is not always achieved, but the effort is always made.

Occupational therapy personnel believe in the value of establishing and supporting rehabilitation services, regardless of how they are funded. Rehabilitation services include those for physical, mental, behavioral, and interpersonal problems. Such rehabilitation services should be available to everyone, not just those who can afford to pay. Occupational therapy personnel work in many countries providing rehabilitation services.

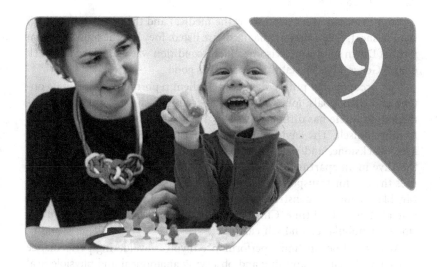

Evaluation, Intervention, and Discharge

The major job functions of occupational therapists and assistants can be broadly summarized into three categories: evaluation, intervention, and discharge. The following case study illustrates how these categories come together in client care.

Joey, a 20-month-old boy with a diagnosis of Down syndrome, is referred by the family pediatrician, Dr. Rodriguez, to a child care center specializing in working with special needs children. The occupational therapist, Erin, will evaluate Joey. The occupational therapy assistant, Mark, can help provide information, but under most state regulatory boards, the occupational therapist holds the primary responsibility for the evaluation process. That process includes three major subcomponents: medical and therapy history, occupational profile, and analysis of occupational performance.

Stein, F., & Reed, K. L.
Occupational Therapy: A Guide for Prospective Students, Consumers, and Advocates (pp. 81-84).
© 2021 Taylor & Francis Group.

Both Erin and Mark can review the medical and therapy history, which is quite short. Joey's age and diagnosis are listed. Joey has the most common form of Down syndrome: trisomy 21. His condition was diagnosed at 1 week of age. General health status is reported as good.

The occupational profile includes the client report, environmental context, and client goals. Joey was referred because he shows signs of developmental delay. He has difficulty crawling, is not walking, and has difficulty feeding himself. The environmental context includes his parents, Mr. and Mrs. Blackstone, and sister, Rosa, age 8 years. According to the address, they live in an apartment about 10 miles from the center. Mrs. Blackstone uses the bus for transportation unless her brother is available to drive her. Mr. Blackstone is a construction worker and often is away from home for extended periods of time. Client goals are to promote developmental milestones in ambulation and self-care.

Analysis of occupational performance involves evaluating performance skills and deficits, examining and observing anatomical and physiological systems in Joey's body that may positively or negatively affect occupational performance, and making note of what contexts or environmental factors may facilitate or hinder performance. Erin begins by observing Joey interact with his mother on the floor of clinic. Joey can sit, but his back looks like a big letter C. He cannot sit with his back straight and head erect. In attempting to crawl, he looks like a baby alligator moving one side of his body and then the other. He has difficulty getting his knees under his hips and shoulders over his hands. As he attempts to pick up some small toy tigers and giraffes, he grabs with all his fingers instead of using his thumb against his index and middle finger. Erin knows that a typically developing child would be able to sit erect at 6 to 7 months, crawl on his hands and knees at 8 to 9 months, walk at about 12 to 13 months, and pick up toys with thumb and fingers at about the same age. Joey is developmentally delayed, as Dr. Rodriguez noted in the referral.

As Erin continues to observe, she notes that Joey's skin color has turned a dusty blue-gray, and his mother lets him rest for a few minutes, saying he is tired. She wonders if he may have a cardiac condition that decreases circulation as activity increases. She makes a note to report the observation to Dr. Rodriguez and ask if Joey has been seen by a cardiologist.

After Joey rests, Erin places the boy in a chair with arms and puts a table with the animal figures in front of him. She takes a bird and pretends to fly it from left to right in front of Joey's eyes to see if they work together to track the bird's path. They do not. One eye tracks to his nose and stays there, while the other eye takes over to watch the bird fly to Joey's right side. Joey may have strabismus, a condition in which the eyes function separately rather than working together as a team. Although Joey cannot report what he sees, the bird may actually appear to drop or rise in its flight pattern because his eyes not only do not track together, but they also do not track in a straight line. Erin notes her observation as another item to report to Dr. Rodriguez. Joey needs a referral to an ophthalmologist to see if surgical correction may be helpful. Note the referral is to an ophthalmologist, a doctor who treats diseases and disorders of the eye, not to an optometrist, who prescribes glasses. Joey may need glasses, but assessment of his possible strabismus should come first.

Next Erin gets a small bowl of applesauce for Joey to eat. She will observe whether Joey is able to use the spoon to scoop up the applesauce, place it in his mouth, and swallow without choking. He is able to perform this task, but Erin does note his large tongue, a problem common in children with Down syndrome. Next, Erin observes that Joey has difficulty grasping Cheerios because he does not have a pincer grasp using his thumb and index finger. This performance deficit had been noted when Joey had difficulty picking up the tiger and giraffe. When Joey does succeed in getting a piece of cereal in his mouth, he does not chew before swallowing, and he chokes as it goes down his throat.

A conversation with Joey's mother about his participation in dressing himself reveals he does not assist in pushing down or pulling up his pants and is not potty-trained. Joey does not speak words, but does make some sounds. His mother also complains that he is a messy eater, often spitting out his food.

While Erin was working with Joey and his mother, Mark was watching some videos about Joey on Mrs. Blackstone's smartphone. Sister Rosa is shown playing with Joey and helping dress and feed him. He also notes another member of the family: a cocker spaniel named Sasha. Joey is shown petting Sasha, grabbing at her fur with his hands, and attempting to follow her around the apartment. Dogs can be good motivators for promoting hand function and ambulation. Mark also observes a couch that could be used to help Joey stand with support and a coffee table to provide opportunity to walk between the two, providing support on both sides. Making use of family, pets, and objects in the home can be useful in developing a home program.

The data from the evaluation can now be assembled for the intervention phase, which will include analyzing the findings, identifying the problems, setting goals, and determining intervention approaches. The findings show Joey is delayed in his motor development. He also needs further assessment by a physical therapist for ambulation and a speech-language pathologist for communication and language skills. An integrated plan of therapy will be needed to address all aspects of the delays noted in the report. Problems identified are ambulation delay including failure to crawl, stand, and walk;

hand grasp delay; difficulty with chewing and swallowing; lack of participation in dressing and undressing; and lack of speech. On the positive side, his mother, sister, and dog can participate in the therapy program.

Setting goals can be based on the problem lists, but also important are the concerns of the parents. Mrs. Blackstone would like the focus of therapy to be on improving feeding skills, dressing skills, and crawling and walking skills. Therefore, the best intervention plan should address these issues. Since transportation is a problem, a home program may work well for Joey. Demonstrations will be needed to show his mother how to facilitate feeding, dressing, and crawling tasks. Videos can be shared to monitor progress. A video and voice program, such as video chat, may be useful to answer immediate questions. Once every 2 weeks, Joey and his mother can return to the clinic or a home visit can be arranged. While Erin must make any changes to the written intervention plan, Mark can assist in monitoring Joey's progress, help identify problems, suggest possible solutions, and participate in clinic or home visits. Erin is also responsible for writing the documentation for the clinic's records, but Mark can provide notes to be included.

Discharge planning is not an immediate concern for Joey, but the long-range plan should be for Joey to attend a preschool program for children with disabilities when he is 3 years old, at least a few hours a day, 5 days a week, to prepare him for school.

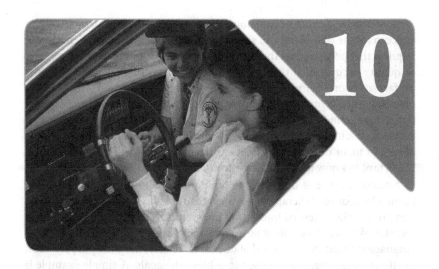

Professional Codes of Ethics

A code of ethics describes the behavior expected of an organization's members. The code of ethics for the American Occupational Therapy Association (AOTA) describes the behavior expected of members who are occupational therapy practitioners, educators, and researchers. The code of ethics for the National Board for Certification in Occupational Therapy (NBCOT) describes behavior expected of occupational therapy personnel certified as registered occupational therapists or certified occupational therapy assistants.

The AOTA Code of Ethics consists of six main principles: beneficence, nonmaleficence, autonomy, justice, veracity, and fidelity. In the context of the code, the word *beneficence* means doing good, *nonmaleficence* means avoiding harm, *autonomy* means self-rule, *justice* means fairness or rightness, *veracity* means truthfulness, and *fidelity* means faithfulness or loyalty. Each word is described here as it appears in the code itself.

Stein, F., & Reed, K. L.
*Occupational Therapy: A Guide for Prospective
Students, Consumers, and Advocates* (pp. 85-88).
© 2021 Taylor & Francis Group.

Beneficence directs occupational therapy personnel to demonstrate a concern for the well-being and safety of the clients being served. Beneficence requires that occupational therapy personnel help others by promoting good or quality occupational therapy services and protecting and defending the welfare of those being served. Services include evaluation, intervention planning, intervention management, documentation, maintaining competency, management and supervision, education or training, and research. Services should be based on the best known information as to what will be of benefit to, or do good for, clients. Current and up-to-date information is important to know and translate into client care.

Nonmaleficence is described as taking actions to refrain from causing harm. Occupational therapy personnel are to abstain from, avoid the risk of, and prevent the potential injury that may result from malicious or harmful intent, unless the good intent outweighs the harm. Nonmaleficence in legal language is called the "standard of due care." That is, the goals pursued must justify the risks that are imposed to achieve the goals. A simple example is that of getting a flu shot. The needle stick may temporarily hurt, but avoiding the flu, which can be fatal, outweighs the temporary pain—the value to life and health exceeds the "cost" of a needle prick. A hospital or other health institution may require occupational therapy personnel to get a flu shot on the basis of preventing potential harm to clients who might contract the flu virus while receiving services from an occupational therapist or assistant who is infected and not vaccinated.

Autonomy has two parts: self-determination and confidentiality. *Self-determination* means the client has the right to accept or refuse occupational therapy, including an evaluation or intervention procedure, and the right to participate in crafting the intervention and discharge plan. In the case of infants, those with intellectual or cognitive disability, or those with dementia, the right may be transferred to parents or guardians. Occupational therapy personnel can encourage the client to participate in occupational therapy programs and explain the potential value of such programs, but cannot force the client to participate. The client has the right to "just say no." *Confidentiality* means the information about a client must be kept private. That is, the information is released only to those people or entities to whom the client has agreed can receive the information. Without the signed agreement, called consent, no information may be shared even with family members or close relatives. Information in paper charts or on computer servers must be kept secure. Client records cannot be carried home in a backpack, saved on a personal computer, or saved to personal cloud space. For more information regarding confidentially, read about the federal law called the Health Insurance Portability and Accountability Act.

Justice also has two parts: procedural and social. *Procedural justice* requires occupational therapy personnel to do what is right as stated in laws, regulations, and policies. Rightness includes graduating from an accredited occupational therapy program, completing the certification examination with a passing score, and obtaining and maintaining a state license. Practitioners, educators, and researchers are all subject to obeying and upholding certain rules, or consequences will be applied. One regulation may concern completing continuing education requirements as a condition for renewing a state licensure. Failure to complete the required number of hours or credits can result in the license being suspended (taken away) for a certain length of time, or the individual being required to complete a certain number of community service hours (free of charge) before the license is restored. During the suspension, the practitioner cannot work or be paid for services provided. *Social justice* is based on nondiscrimination, fairness, and equality. In occupational therapy, social justice means that services are provided to all people, regardless of the type of disability, socioeconomic status, ethnic background, sexual orientation, religion, or other means by which society divides people into groups in which some may be viewed as more worthy than others. During World War I, for example, occupational therapy services were provided to all servicemen and servicewomen regardless of their rank. The private and the general were treated the same, based not on their rank in the U.S. military, but on their needs for occupational therapy.

Veracity requires occupational therapy personnel to provide accurate, objective, and comprehensive information when representing the profession of occupational therapy. Keeping it real starts with preparing and presenting a resume that accurately and honestly states credentials, qualifications, education, experience, training, roles, duties, competence, and contributions when applying for a position in occupational therapy. Truthfulness continues with writing objective reports on the evaluation and assessment of a client; stating realistic goals in an intervention plan; writing notes accurately about the progress, or lack of progress, for a client's permanent record; and preparing a client for discharge. Accurate communication should also be provided to colleagues, administrators, and payers, such as insurance companies. Veracity also applies to advertising and marketing, which should state realistic expectations. A person with a serious spinal cord and brain injury, for example, is unlikely to be running a marathon race next month. Be honest, accurate, and objective.

Fidelity requires occupational therapy personnel to treat clients, colleagues, and other professionals with respect, discretion, and integrity. It requires commitment, faithfulness, and loyalty to fulfill the duties and responsibilities that the occupational therapist or assistant agreed to do when accepting the job. Equally important is that fidelity requires that occupational therapy personnel not say disparaging remarks or act in a manner that disrespects clients, colleagues, other professionals, or institutions. Fidelity is most often an issue in communications that can be retrieved, including posts on social media, all computer-based formats, and printed media, including letters or class assignments. Occupational therapy practitioners may encounter clients whom they do not consider easy to treat. Educators find some students more likable than others. Researchers find some research subjects more cooperative than others. Unless they are self-employed, everybody has an opinion about the boss. The issue is how the displeasure is expressed. If incompetent, unethical, or illegal actions are observed, the actions should be reported to the proper authorities but not broadcast for the world to hear. Reportable actions include experiencing harassment or observing behavior that is impaired due to abuse of alcohol, pain killers, or other drug or substance misuse. The focus of fidelity should be on preserving, respecting, and safeguarding reputations and resources.

The AOTA Code of Ethics applies to all of its members. Serious violations may result in loss of membership, but not necessarily the license to practice. However, if the state licensure board that regulates occupational therapy practice has adopted the AOTA Code of Ethics, code violations may result in sanctions, including the loss of the license to practice. Knowing about and abiding by the Code of Ethics is important to maintaining professional standards of conduct.

The NBCOT Code of Conduct covers the same six topics as the AOTA Code of Ethics, but the organization focuses primarily on justice and veracity related to the certification process. Coverage of beneficence, nonmaleficence, autonomy, and fidelity is likewise directed to concerns related to certification and also to the NBCOT as an organization. Signing up to take the certification examination also means agreeing to abide by the NBCOT Code of Conduct.

State licensure boards may create their own set of ethics statements. Consulting the state rules and regulations for occupational therapy will inform the reader as to what ethics statements apply in that state.

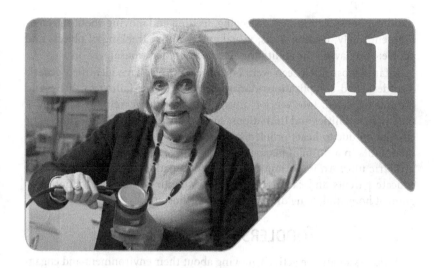

Occupational Therapy Clients

Occupational therapists work with people of all ages to promote function, occupational performance, and participation in everyday activities. Although the purpose remains the same, the occupations and activities change with age, developmental abilities, acute conditions, and chronic diseases. Examples of what occupational therapists do with clients of different ages and abilities are presented in this chapter.

PREMATURE AND AT-RISK NEONATES (1 TO 12 MONTHS)

The focus of occupational therapy for infants is on promoting sensory-motor development in sequence. This includes raising the head from a bed or table, propping oneself on hands and elbows, rolling over, sitting up, and

Stein, F., & Reed, K. L.
Occupational Therapy: A Guide for Prospective Students, Consumers, and Advocates (pp. 89-94).
© 2021 Taylor & Francis Group.

standing; best positioning for sleeping, feeding and moving about the environment safely; feeding skills; visual and auditory tracking of objects and people; and having the ability to calm oneself after arousal.

Infants most often seen were born prematurely, have identified genetic disorders, had complications during delivery, or are failing to thrive and grow as expected. Intervention always begins with a careful assessment of the infant's abilities and limitations, such as breathing difficulties and poor circulation due to heart problems. Practitioners usually work directly with the infants in a hospital neonatal intensive care unit, newborn nursery, or pediatric unit. An important part of the occupational therapy service is to educate parents and caregivers on how to continue the intervention program at home following discharge from the hospital.

TODDLERS (1 TO 3 YEARS)

Toddlers should be actively moving about their environment and engaging in self-care and play activities. Toddlers referred to occupational therapy include those who were born with abnormalities in their bone, muscles, and joints; acquired a brain injury from a fall or vehicle accident; lost abilities following a disease of the nervous system; have sensory losses in vision or other sensory systems; or exhibit behavioral disorders, such as autism. Occupational therapy intervention will be more varied because the range of deficits and dysfunction is wider. Skills may include self-feeding, pushing down and pulling up pants, achieving eye-hand coordination, demonstrating thumb-finger skills, holding and transferring objects between hands, continuing to improve motor skills, increasing communication skills, and developing social skills. Practitioners may be employed by an independently owned clinic, or a facility designed for special needs children and sponsored by a hospital or other health care service. As with infants, an important part of the occupational therapy service is to educate parents and caregivers on how to continue the intervention program at home.

PRESCHOOLERS (4 TO 5 YEARS)

Preschoolers should be engaged in self-care, sensorimotor, learning, communication, and social activities. Preschoolers referred to occupational therapy usually have developmental delays in attaining age-appropriate skills. Occupational therapy intervention is focused on evaluating the areas of developmental delay (i.e., motor, sensory, cognitive, perceptual, and social) and the environmental factors (i.e., family members, living situation, finances, and community resources) available to aid in carrying out an intervention program. Intervention may include the addition of assistive devices, such as a wheelchair, special computer programs, or other modified equipment to facilitate performance. Although play and fun activities continue to be used in intervention programs, learning activities that involve group interaction may be introduced. Practitioners may be employed by an independently owned clinic, a school-based program, or a state-sponsored program designed for disabled children. The intervention program should include family and caregivers in all goals and the methods used to obtain the goals. Home visits or the use of video are useful to evaluate needs and monitor progress.

ELEMENTARY SCHOOL CHILDREN (6 TO 10 YEARS)

Most children with disabilities are able to attend school, although their level of participation in the basic curriculum may vary from very limited to full engagement. The role of the occupational therapy practitioner is to facilitate participation and engagement in the learning and educational activities the school system offers. Practitioners are not substitute teachers, but instead work cooperatively with teachers to maximize the teaching-learning environment for each child. Examples might include using specialized computer software programs, modifying a chair to provide better seating and positioning for working at a desk or table, decreasing the amount of light and sound to reduce distractions in the environment, changing the placement of the child's work area to reduce social interaction during time devoted to individualized seatwork lessons, or recommending specialized learning programs that are developed especially for disabled children and that are not known to the teacher. Practitioners may be employed by a school district or be contract employees who are paid by a hospital or other health care organization. Occupational therapy practitioners working in school settings usually do not provide rehabilitation services designed to directly reduce the disability or dysfunction. Such rehabilitation services are usually provided by hospitals or clinics not associated with the school system. School-based practitioners may interact with the therapy personnel from such hospitals or clinics, especially if significant changes are made to the child's rehabilitation program as might occur after a surgery procedure.

MIDDLE SCHOOLERS AND HIGH SCHOOLERS (11 TO 17 YEARS)

Preteens and teenagers with disabilities who are in middle or high school grades usually have been seen for several years. Typically, the occupational therapy practitioner is monitoring the child to determine if changes are needed to continue maximum participation. Examples might include consulting with teachers unfamiliar with the child or types of modifications needed to facilitate learning, and making recommendations that enable the child to move about the environment safely, such as moving in the cafeteria or from one classroom to another. High school buildings may have multiple floors, which can present a challenge for a child in a wheelchair to get to different classrooms located on more than one level. Modifications in the schedule or use of an elevator may be necessary, even if the elevator is not normally available to students.

Another example is the implementation of a transitional living program designed to help students with disabilities learn the skills needed to live and work in the community after graduation or the end of school-age eligibility at 18 or 21 years, depending on the state policy. Methods may include learning to manage time, creating and keeping a budget, using public transportation, and doing household chores. Practitioners may be employed by the school district or be contracted from a local or state health service agency. Practitioners who work with preteens and teenagers need to include them fully in any intervention program because their willingness to participate in the program will largely determine its failure or success.

YOUNG ADULTS (18 TO 44 YEARS)

Occupational therapy services for young adults most often involve acute changes in ability to function. Brain and spinal cord injuries may occur due to vehicle accidents, gunshot injuries, sports activities, or accidental falls. Mental health disorders may include substance abuse and addiction (e.g., alcohol, opioids, heroin, or other narcotics), severe depression, manic episodes, schizophrenia, or other behavioral disorders.

Typically, occupational therapy practitioners are employed in hospitals providing acute care and outpatient clinics providing continuing care. The focus of intervention is to help the person regain function and occupational performance in the skills of everyday living, including activities of daily living, work, and leisure. Rehabilitation may require methods to address motor, perceptual, cognitive, and social deficits. Acute care facilities often focus on helping clients regain activities of daily living, including self-care skills. However, programs for mental health disorders usually focus on daily living tasks associated with creating and maintaining a time schedule, budgeting income and expenses, locating and applying for work, getting a driver's license or using public transportation, shopping at a grocery store, and performing household tasks, such as preparing healthful foods. Some cases may require modifications to the home or work situation to facilitate access to the building and increase the person's ability to perform work tasks within the building.

MIDDLE-AGED ADULTS (45 TO 64 YEARS)

Individuals who are middle-aged may experience the same injuries and disorders as younger adults, but in addition, are more likely to incur dysfunction from chronic disorders as well. Examples may include arthritis, limiting joint movement and causing pain; obesity from unhealthful diets; type 2 diabetes resulting in loss of sensation in the feet as well as visual problems, stroke, or other cardiac conditions; Parkinson's disease; multiple sclerosis; and cancer. Although the focus of intervention continues to be to help the person regain function and occupational performance, management of chronic conditions requires consideration to making adjustments to the living environment and maintaining as much function as possible. A portion of the intervention plan may be devoted to modifying the home to increase safety and introducing devices to make tasks easier to perform. Practitioners are employed in hospitals and outpatient clinics, but in addition, some may be working in nursing homes that provide rehabilitation services or providing home care. Rehabilitation methods should address the individual, but also address the situation in which the person lives and works to improve ability to perform desired or required tasks.

OLDER ADULTS (65 TO 79 YEARS)

Older adults may experience any of the conditions as young and middle-aged adults, but chronic conditions are more often in evidence. Cognitive dysfunction may occur, including memory loss due to Alzheimer's disease or other dementias. Depressive episodes may occur as the person feels increasingly useless and worthless, especially if retirement has not been well-planned so that other activities take the place of paid work tasks. Older adults are more likely to fall and break a hip or other bones. The process of aging alone causes dysfunction. When the aging process is added to one or more chronic conditions, the degree or level of dysfunction often increases. Maintaining maximum function of the body and mind continues to be an important goal, but use of adaptive devices and modifications of the home and community environment becomes equally as important. Alternative

environments, such as assisted living or nursing care facilities, may be considered. Practitioners working in hospitals may see clients of any age, but
those working in skilled nursing homes or long-term care facilities may see
older adults most of the time. Rehabilitation methods should address the
individual but also focus on the home environment, such as a house, apartment, nursing care facility, or other living arrangement.

VERY OLD ADULTS (80 YEARS AND OLDER)

Very old adults usually experience dysfunction due to existing chronic
conditions and the aging process but may experience additional dysfunction due to an acute episode, such as a fall, stroke, or surgery. Feelings of
hopelessness and being useless or worthless may increase and may interfere
with the interest in regaining performance of everyday living occupations.
Although self-care skills in eating, dressing, and grooming decrease caregiver burden, the individual may need to focus first on regaining the ability
to perform a valued leisure activity, such as playing a game, taking care of
the plants, attending a religious service, or going to a sports activity. When
the valued activity is achieved, performing self-care skills takes on meaning
and purpose, and the effort to perform the tasks is more willingly assumed.
Practitioners working with very old adults are more likely to be employed
by skilled nursing homes or long-term care facilities, or to be providing
home care services. Modifying the occupation to be performed and the
environment in which the occupation occurs becomes more important as
the individual's ability to adapt to the occupational and environmental
demands decreases.

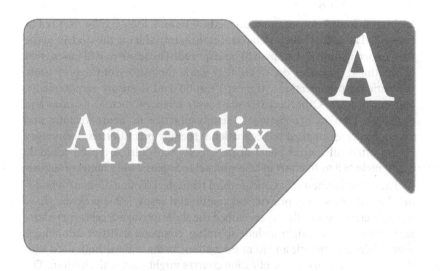

What Is It Like to Be an Occupational Therapy Student?

TRADITIONAL IN-CLASS PROGRAM

Potential students often ask what it is like to be an occupational therapy student in a traditional program where students attend class at the college or university. In other words, what the student will be learning and doing per week and semester. Although there is no single answer, there is a general profile. The first semester or trimester of the occupational therapy program requires learning many new words, phrases, and terminology as the student masters the language of medicine in general and the lingo of occupational therapy specifically. An example is the *Occupational Therapy Practice Framework*, which is updated every 5 years. The *Occupational Therapy Practice Framework* includes a list of words and definitions in the glossary of terms. All students must learn those words forward and sometimes

Stein, F., & Reed, K. L.
Occupational Therapy: A Guide for Prospective Students, Consumers, and Advocates (pp. 95-98).
© 2021 Taylor & Francis Group.

backward. In addition, a course on medical terminology may be required or embedded as part of another course. Lectures introducing the student to the field of occupational therapy will be required. The lectures will cover what occupational therapists do, where they work, the history of the profession, the national organizations, the certification and licensure requirements, and much more. Other lectures may cover sciences, such as diseases and disorders, seen in occupational therapy practice or neuroanatomy and neurophysiology applied to occupational therapy practitioners. Laboratory classes often fill several hours of the weekly schedule. A typical schedule might include 8 to 10 hours of laboratory classes plus 9 to 12 hours of lecture.

The second semester (second or third trimester) is often devoted to building the skills needed to practice occupational therapy. Some programs have separate classes on skills, others embed the skills into age-level theory classes. Separate classes might include splinting, computer assistive technology, adapted devices, muscle and joint evaluation, media and methods used with children, etc. Theory and application courses might start with children. The course might cover the assessment instruments used to evaluate occupational performance problems in children, how to develop an occupational profile and plan of intervention, examples of intervention programs, and how to document progress and plan for discharge and follow-up. Lecture and laboratory courses would continue. The number of hours in laboratory classes often continues to exceed the number of lecture hours. Lecture classes may include projects, such as planning an occupation-based program for clients with opioid addition. Laboratory classes may include projects, such as planning and conducting a group activity for five older adults average age 72 years (note that the older adults may be fellow students role-playing as older adults), making a splint for a hand or wrist injury, or adapting a toy to allow it to be operated remotely for a child with limited mobility. Laboratory classes may also require periodic competency testing in which the student must demonstrate the ability to perform a certain task, such as transfering a client with poor balance safely from chair to bed and back, evaluating a client's need for a wheelchair and providing exact measurements so the wheelchair fits the client correctly, or instructing a client on how to put on socks using a sock aid.

The second year (third and fourth semesters) continues the theory and application of occupational therapy practice. Classes cover the role and function of occupational therapy with young adults, people who are middle-aged, and older individuals. The focus is on evaluation, planning, intervention, and discharge. Observation in real clinics and facilities is often included. Practice in documentation or writing progress notes is provided. Understanding legal requirements and ethical practice is included. Opportunity for elective classes may be available, but the subject matter may be restricted to topics related to occupational therapy practice, education, or research. Lectures and laboratory time may be combined. Student may feel they spend most of their time in laboratory classes because practice in skill development and application of media and methods is critical to becoming a competent practitioner.

An important element in understanding the occupational therapy program is its relatively fixed schedule. In general, students need to be prepared to complete the courses in sequence within the school calendar. Occupational therapy courses are usually offered only one time per year and may be bundled together so that all must be taken together in a given semester or trimester. The option to pick and choose which classes to take and when to take them is usually not available. Likewise the time of day may be fixed. If the student plans to work while enrolled in the occupational therapy program, the work schedule will need to be flexible or limited to hours when classes are not scheduled, such as on weekends. Missing classes because of work assignments may result in failing a class. Because the classes are in sequence and offered on a limited schedule, failure in one class may cause the student to have to add another full year to the schedule of completing the course requirements to graduate and establish the requirement to take the certification examination. Occupational therapy student needs to prioritize school and class attendance over work hours. Occupational therapy education is a hands-on, demonstration, and practice discipline. If your hands (and head) are not in class, you are not learning the knowledge, skills, and attitudes necessary to become a competent occupational therapy practitioner.

ONLINE CLASSES

Some occupational therapy educational programs offer online classes as well as in-person onsite attendance classes. In the time of coronavirus (COVID-19) in 2020, many occupational therapy classes moved online. Online courses work well for lecture material. Learning factual knowledge via computer programs can be efficient and effective. The schedule of classes is often more flexible and may be available in the evening or on weekends. Costs may be less since the student does not need transportation to attend in person or pay for parking if driving a vehicle. Weather conditions outside generally do not affect the computer inside unless the power goes out. The disadvantage of online lecture courses is the face-to-face contact with other students and the instructor. Occupational therapy students learn from each other both in class and in the informal exchanges that occur between classes. Another major disadvantage of online classes is that they do not work well for laboratory or hands-on classes. Therefore, some occupational therapy educational programs are actually hybrids. That is, some lecture courses are available online, but the laboratory classes require in-person and onsite attendance. Attendance may be required on a weekly basis. Other arrangements may require the student to come to campus two to four times a semester or trimester for a concentrated time, such as 3 days (Friday to Sunday) for classes scheduled 6 to 8 hours per day. The concentrated schedule includes practice time and checkout for competency testing.

Potential students need to evaluate their preferred learning style. Some students enjoy learning via computer and do not mind having to sit in front of a computer to learn subject material. Other students do not enjoy learning via computer and prefer the face-to-face contact with other students and faculty. Still others are able to accommodate both computer-based classes and in-person onsite classes. The choice of an occupational therapy education program should be based, in part, on the student's analysis of their preferred learning style.

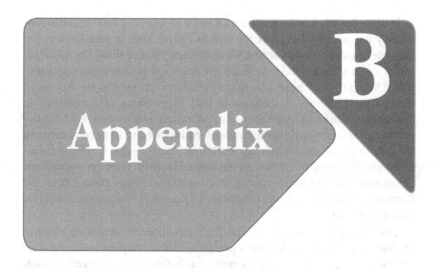

State and Jurisdiction Regulation of Occupational Therapy

The licensure to practice occupational therapy is controlled in each state and jurisdiction (Washington, DC, Guam, and Puerto Rico) by a regulatory board. Board membership differs depending on the state or jurisdiction. Some members are appointed while others may be elected. Their job is to write, revise, and enforce the rules and regulations that enact the state or jurisdiction law passed by the legislators. The document that includes the rules and regulations is available online, but the title may vary. A typical title is "Occupational Therapy Rules" or "Occupational Therapy Practice Act and Rules" plus the name of the state or jurisdiction. Note that the rules and regulations are usually a separate document from the law that created the occupational therapy licensure act. The law established the legal framework within the state or jurisdiction system of governance but does not spell out the details about the provision of occupational therapy services. Those details are the purview of the rules and regulations.

Stein, F., & Reed, K. L.
Occupational Therapy: A Guide for Prospective Students, Consumers, and Advocates (pp. 99-101).
© 2021 Taylor & Francis Group.

Within the rules is information of value in learning how occupational therapy is governed and practiced within a given state or jurisdiction. For example, the definition of occupational therapy practice should be included, which states what media or methods are approved in that state or jurisdiction. The details may be similar to the definition approved by the American Occupational Therapy Association in 2011 (Appendix C) but may include or exclude some items. Another useful definition is the one that defines the practice of occupational therapy and determines who must have a license in the state or jurisdiction. Occupational therapy personnel may refer to themselves as a clinician, practitioner, educator, consultant, manager, supervisor, instructor, professor, or researcher. Are any of these titles exempt from the licensure requirement or must everyone be licensed? The answer should be stated in the rules.

The rules should also include specific instructions for obtaining a license in that state. For example, can a person obtain a temporary license after completing the academic requirements but before taking the certification examination? What about a person who holds a valid license in another state? Can the license holder obtain a temporary license or must a permanent license be obtained before the person can work as an occupational therapist or assistant in that state or jurisdiction? There should also be a section in the rules that explains how to renew a license, including details of continuing education requirements, if any.

Another useful section of the rules should describe the supervision requirements between occupational therapy supervisor and occupational therapy assistants. For example, what tasks can be delegated to the occupational therapy assistant versus the tasks that must be performed by an occupational therapist? Must all notes entered into the client's permanent record or chart be cosigned by the occupational therapy supervisor or can the note be signed by the occupational therapy assistant alone? How many occupational therapy assistants can be supervised by one occupational therapist? According to the rules, how often must the occupational therapy supervisor meet face-to-face with the occupational therapy assistant or assistants being supervised? All of these questions should be addressed in the rules or in a section of frequently asked questions.

A third section of interest should explain the provision of occupational therapy services recognized under the rules. For example, is a referral (or script) needed from a physician for any client seen in occupational therapy, or are there exceptions? Exceptions might include conditions that are not considered medical conditions, such as a child with attention deficit hyperactivity disorder, a consultation to modify a home for better access and safety, or the preparation of general purpose instruction materials based on occupational therapy methods. Some rules are written to provide exceptions, but some permit no exceptions; all clients seen in occupational therapy must have a referral. A related issue is when the referral must be received. Some rules are written to state that an evaluation (screening, consultation, or monitoring) may be performed by an occupational therapist without a referral. If the client does not qualify for occupational therapy services or refuses to accept the intervention plan of care, no referral will be needed. If, however, the client agrees to participate and attend appointments, then a request for a referral can be initiated. Note that evaluation services must be performed by the occupational therapist, although the occupational therapy assistant can provide data. The rules may also state whether an evaluation must be performed face-to-face or may be conducted via electronic methods, such as telehealth. In states with large rural areas, telehealth, or other information technologies, can substantially increase the reach of occupational therapy services to those who live many miles from the physical location of the hospital, clinic, or school. In addition, the rules should provide explanations for who is responsible for developing and revising the plan of care, which practitioner is responsible for writing reports to document that services have been provided, and who is responsible for discharging clients or discontinuing occupational therapy services.

A fourth section of interest may be the one that describes the disciplinary actions that can be implemented if license holders do not follow the rules. States and jurisdictions have a wide choice of disciplinary actions depending on how severe the rule infraction is determined to be. Lesser disciplinary actions might include a letter of reprimand, a fine of $500 or less, or a requirement to complete a designated number of hours of community service. More severe infractions may result in a requirement to complete a specific number of continuing education hours, sign up and complete a rehabilitation program, such as a drug treatment program, or the suspension of the license to practice for several months. For very severe infractions, such as repeated failure to complete the requirements specified in previous disciplinary actions or endangering the lives of clients, the license may be removed permanently and the person may be referred to law enforcement personnel for criminal prosecution.

Finally, a section should be identified that states the current fees to obtain an initial license and renewal plus any special fees for additional services. Fees, of course, can be increased yearly, so the current fee schedule might change if a student does not intend to graduate from an occupational therapy program and complete the certification examination for several years from now. Nevertheless, the fee schedule gives a working estimate of the costs to be incurred to become a licensed practitioner in occupational therapy in the state or jurisdiction.

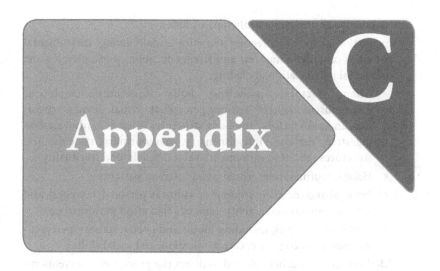

Appendix C

Definition of Occupational Therapy

The practice of occupational therapy means the therapeutic use of occupations, including everyday life activities with individuals, groups, populations, or organizations to support participation, performance, and function in roles and situations in homes, schools, workplaces, communities, and other settings. Occupational therapy services are provided for habilitation, rehabilitation, and the promotion of health and wellness to those who have or are at risk for developing an illness, injury, disease, disorder, condition, impairment, disability, activity limitation, or participation restriction. Occupational therapy addresses the physical, cognitive, psychosocial, sensory-perceptual, and other aspects of performance in a variety of contexts and environments to support engagement in occupations that affect physical and mental health, well-being, and quality of life.

Stein, F., & Reed, K. L.
Occupational Therapy: A Guide for Prospective
Students, Consumers, and Advocates (pp. 103-105).
© 2021 Taylor & Francis Group.

The practice of occupational therapy includes:

- Evaluation of factors affecting activities of daily living, instrumental activities of daily living, rest and sleep, education, work, play, leisure, and social participation, including:
  - Client factors, including body functions (such as neuromusculoskeletal, sensory-perceptual, visual, mental, cognitive, and pain factors) and body structures (such as cardiovascular, digestive, nervous, integumentary, genitourinary systems, and structures related to movement), values, beliefs, and spirituality
  - Habits, routines, roles, rituals, and behavior patterns
  - Physical and social environments, cultural, personal, temporal, and virtual contexts and activity demands that affect performance
  - Performance skills, including motor and praxis, sensory-perceptual, emotional, cognitive, communication, and social skills
- Methods or approaches selected to direct the process of interventions, such as:
  - Establishment, remediation, or restoration of a skill or ability that has not yet developed, is impaired, or is in decline
  - Compensation, modification, or adaptation of activity or environment to enhance performance or to prevent injuries, disorders, or other conditions
  - Retention and enhancement of skills or abilities without which performance in everyday life activities would decline
  - Promotion of health and wellness, including the use of self-management strategies, to enable or enhance performance in everyday life activities
  - Prevention of barriers to performance and participation, including injury and disability prevention
- Interventions and procedures to promote or enhance safety and performance in activities of daily living, instrumental activities of daily living, rest and sleep, education, work, play, leisure, and social participation, including:
  - Therapeutic use of occupations, exercises, and activities
  - Training in self-care, self-management, health management and maintenance, home management, community/reintegration, and school activities and work performance
  - Development, remediation, or compensation of neuromusculoskeletal, sensory-perceptual, visual, mental, and cognitive functions, pain tolerance and management and behavioral skills

o Therapeutic use of self, including one's personality, insights, perceptions, and judgment, as part of the therapeutic process

o Education and training of individuals, including family members, caregivers, groups, populations, and others

o Care coordination, case management, and transition services

o Consultative services to groups, programs, organizations, or communities

o Modification of environments (home, work, school, or community) and adaptation of processes, including the application of ergonomic principles

o Assessment, design, fabrication, application, fitting, and training in seating and positions, assistive technology, adaptive devices, and orthotic devices, and training in the use of prosthetic devices

o Assessment, recommendation, and training in techniques to enhance functional mobility, including management of wheelchairs and other mobility devices

o Low vision rehabilitation

o Driver rehabilitation and community mobility

o Management of feeding, eating, and swallowing to enable eating and feeding performance

o Application of physical agent modalities and use of a range of specific therapeutic procedures (such as wound care management, intervention to enhance sensory-perceptual and cognitive processing, and manual therapy) to enhance performance skills

o Facilitating the occupational performance of groups, populations, or organizations through the modification of environments and adaption of processes

Note: Items were changed from numbers to bullets to avoid appearing to rank order the importance of any given item.

Adopted by the American Occupational Therapy Association Representative Assembly 4/14/11 (Agenda A13, Charge 18)

Reprinted with permission from American Occupational Therapy Association.

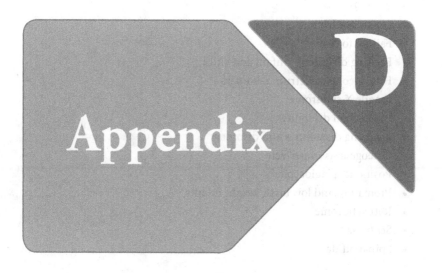

Appendix D

List of Diagnoses and Conditions Seen in Occupational Therapy

DEVELOPMENTAL DISORDERS

- Arthrogryposis multiplex congenita
- Asperger syndrome
- Attention deficit/hyperactivity disorder
- Autism and autistic spectrum disorders
- Brachial plexus birth injuries
- Cerebral palsy
- Child abuse/maltreatment
- Developmental coordination disorder
- Developmental delay—child
- Developmental disabilities—adolescent and adult

Stein, F., & Reed, K. L.
*Occupational Therapy: A Guide for Prospective
Students, Consumers, and Advocates* (pp. 107-112).
© 2021 Taylor & Francis Group.

- Down syndrome
- Failure to thrive
- Feeding disorders—infant and child
- Fetal alcohol spectrum disorders
- Fragile X syndrome
- Intellectual disability
- Learning disabilities and disorders
- Osteogenesis imperfecta
- Positional plagiocephaly
- Premature and low birth weight infants
- Rett syndrome
- Scoliosis
- Spinal bifida

SENSORY DISORDERS

- Age-related macular degeneration
- Agnosia
- Ayres sensory integration dysfunction
- Back pain
- Benign paroxysmal positional vertigo
- Blindness and visual impairment
- Body image disturbance
- Body scheme disorders
- Chronic pain
- Complex regional pain syndrome
- Deafness and hearing loss
- Low vision
- Sensory defensiveness
- Sensory discrimination disorder
- Sensory integration dysfunction
- Sensory modulation dysfunction
- Sensory processing disorders
- Sensory processing patterns (Dunn's model)
- Vestibular disorders
- Visual deficits in stroke and brain injury
- Visual-perceptual dysfunction

NERVOUS SYSTEM DISORDERS

- Amyotrophic lateral sclerosis
- Coma, stupor, and vegetative states
- Cubital tunnel syndrome
- Guillain-Barré syndrome
- Hemiplegia in stroke and brain injury
- Huntington's disease
- Multiple sclerosis
- Parkinson's disease
- Post-poliomyelitis syndrome
- Radial tunnel syndrome
- Seizure disorders
- Stroke/cerebral vascular accident
- Swallowing disorders—adult

CARDIOPULMONARY DISORDERS

- Chronic obstructive pulmonary disease
- Heart disease and myocardial infraction

HAND AND WRIST CONDITIONS

- Arthritis of the hand and wrist
- Arthroplasty—hand
- Boutonniere deformity
- Carpal tunnel syndrome
- Cumulative trauma disorders
- De Quervain's disease
- Dupuytren's contracture
- Edema of the hand and upper extremity
- Extensor tendon injuries
- Finger fractures
- Flexor tendon injuries
- Mallet finger
- Osteoarthritis of the thumb

- Swan neck deformity
- Thumb injuries and conditions
- Trigger finger

INJURIES

- Amputation—upper and lower extremity
- Arthroplasty—hip and knee
- Athletic injuries—upper extremity
- Brain injuries
- Fractures—radius, elbow, and hip
- Lateral epicondylitis
- Peripheral nerve injuries—upper extremity
- Replantation of the hand and arm
- Rotator cuff injury
- Spinal cord injuries
- Tenolysis
- Upper extremity injuries to musicians and artists

MUSCULOSKELETAL DISORDERS

- Fibromyalgia
- Frozen shoulder
- Joint stiffness
- Juvenile rheumatoid arthritis
- Muscular dystrophies
- Musculoskeletal disorders
- Osteoarthritis
- Osteoporosis
- Rheumatoid arthritis

SYSTEMIC DISORDERS

- Chronic fatigue syndrome
- Diabetes mellitus
- Incontinence
- Renal disease and renal failure
- Scleroderma
- Systemic lupus erythematosus

IMMUNOLOGIC AND INFECTIOUS DISEASES

- Acquired immunodeficiency syndrome/human immunodeficiency virus
- Allergies and asthma
- Cancer/neoplasms
- Lymphedema

SKIN DISORDERS

- Burns
- Pressure ulcers
- Scars
- Wound care

COGNITIVE-PERCEPTUAL DISORDERS

- Alzheimer's disease
- Apraxia
- Cognitive disability/dysfunction—brain injury and stroke
- Dementia
- Executive dysfunction
- Impaired self-awareness
- Unilateral neglect

MENTAL DISORDERS

- Anxiety
- Bipolar disorders
- Depression—primary and secondary
- Eating disorders
- Emotion disturbance/behavior disorders—child and adolescent
- Forensic occupational therapy (prisons)
- Personality disorders
- Post-traumatic stress disorder
- Schizophrenia
- Substance abuse, dependence, and addiction
- Suicide and suicidal behavior

LIFESTYLE DISORDERS

- Driving—older adult or after neurological impairment
- Elder abuse and elder self-neglect
- Falls
- Homelessness
- Loss, grief, and bereavement
- Obesity and overweight
- Refugees, asylum seekers, immigrants, and displaced persons
- Sleep and wakefulness disorders
- Terminal and life-threatening illness
- Violence

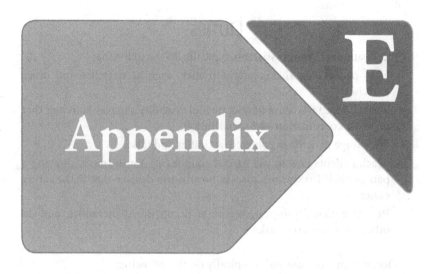

Appendix E

What Occupational Therapy Assistants and Aides Do

Occupational therapy aides may handle some clerical tasks, such as answering calls from patients and scheduling appointments.

Occupational therapy assistants and aides help patients develop, recover, improve, as well as maintain the skills needed for daily living and working. Occupational therapy assistants are directly involved in providing therapy to patients; occupational therapy aides typically perform support activities. Both assistants and aides work under the direction of occupational therapists.

Stein, F., & Reed, K. L.
Occupational Therapy: A Guide for Prospective Students, Consumers, and Advocates (pp. 113-115).
© 2021 Taylor & Francis Group.

DUTIES

Occupational therapy assistants typically do the following:

- Help patients do therapeutic activities, such as stretches and other exercises
- Lead children who have developmental disabilities in play activities that promote coordination and socialization
- Encourage patients to complete activities and tasks
- Teach patients how to use special equipment—for example, showing a patient with Parkinson's disease how to use devices that make eating easier
- Record patients' progress, report to occupational therapists, and do other administrative tasks

Occupational therapy aides typically do the following:

- Prepare treatment areas, such as setting up therapy equipment
- Transport patients
- Clean treatment areas and equipment
- Help patients with billing and insurance forms
- Perform clerical tasks, including scheduling appointments and answering telephones

Occupational therapy assistants collaborate with occupational therapists to develop and carry out a treatment plan for each patient. Plans include diverse activities such as teaching the proper way for patients to move from a bed into a wheelchair and advising patients on the best way to stretch their muscles. For example, an occupational therapy assistant might work with injured workers to help them get back into the workforce by teaching them how to work around lost motor skills. Occupational therapy assistants also may work with people who have learning disabilities, teaching them skills that allow them to be more independent.

Assistants monitor activities to make sure that patients are doing them correctly. They record the patient's progress and provide feedback to the occupational therapist so that the therapist can change the treatment plan if the patient is not getting the desired results.

Occupational therapy aides typically prepare materials and assemble equipment used during treatment. They may assist patients with moving to and from treatment areas. After a therapy session, aides clean the treatment area, put away equipment, and gather laundry.

Occupational therapy aides fill out insurance forms and other paperwork and are responsible for a range of clerical tasks, such as scheduling appointments, answering the telephone, and monitoring inventory levels.

Adapted from Bureau of Labor Statistics, U. S. Department of Labor. *Occupational outlook handbook: Occupational therapy assistants and aides.* https://www.bls.gov/ooh/healthcare/occupational-therapy-assistants-and-aides.htm

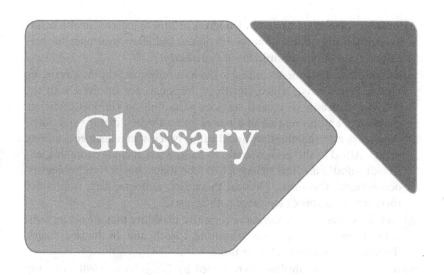

Glossary

activities of daily living: Tasks that are essential for self-care, such as bathing, grooming, dressing, feeding, transferring from bed to wheelchair, and toileting.

activity analysis: An essential part of what the occupational therapist does in sequencing activities or tasks so that they fit the needs of an individual. Through this process, the occupational therapist breaks down the steps in performing an activity, such as in cooking, using public transportation, or applying for a job.

adaptive equipment: Self-help devices that enable an individual with a disability to engage in showering by using a bench and grab bars, in grooming by using a long-handled bath brush, in dressing by using elastic laces, in feeding by using a spork (spoon and fork), and in toileting by using a raised toilet seat.

Stein, F., & Reed, K. L.
*Occupational Therapy: A Guide for Prospective
Students, Consumers, and Advocates* (pp. 117-122).
© 2021 Taylor & Francis Group.

Affordable Care Act: Enacted by Congress in 2010 to increase health insurance, lower premiums, improve efficiency, and allow insurance for pre-existing conditions for millions of Americans.

allied health profession: According to the Association of Schools Advancing Health Professions, "Allied Health professionals are involved with the delivery of health or related services pertaining to the identification, evaluation, and prevention of diseases and disorders; dietary and nutrition services; rehabilitation and health systems management, among others. Allied health professionals, to name a few, include dental hygienists, diagnostic medical sonographers, dietitians, medical technologists, occupational therapists, physical therapists, radiographers, respiratory therapists, and speech language pathologists."

Alzheimer's disease: A progressive cognitive disability that affects an individual's memory, judgement, reasoning, speech, and, in the later stages, the ability to perform self-care tasks.

Americans with Disabilities Act: Passed by Congress in 1990 to ensure people with disabilities do not face job discrimination and do have handicapped access to buildings and communication.

aphasia: Disability occurring because of brain damage that affects speech.

assistive technology: According to federal guidelines, "An assistive technology device is defined as 'any item, piece of equipment, or product system, whether acquired commercially off the shelf, modified, or customized, that is used to increase, maintain, or improve functional capabilities of a child with a disability'." This definition can also be applied to devices for adults with disabilities.

audiologist: A health care and rehabilitation professional who evaluates and treats individuals with hearing disorders. A master's degree is required for licensure and practice.

autism: A disability associated with childhood, with symptoms that involve withdrawal from social relationships, language disturbances, and behavioral problems. The symptoms can be mild, moderate, or severe.

behavior therapy: Interventions based on learning theory using positive reinforcements or disincentives.

biofeedback techniques: Intervention techniques to help clients achieve goals, such as controlling symptoms through meditation and relaxation.

carpal tunnel syndrome: Symptoms of pain and numbness in the hand from work-related repetitive motion injuries.

cerebral palsy: Usually caused by a birth injury and resulting in cognitive and sensory/motor disabilities.

certified occupational therapist: Certified occupational therapists work under the supervision of registered occupational therapists to implement therapy programs and interventions.

complementary and alternative medicine: Interventions, such as acupuncture, tai chi, yoga, and herbal remedies, that are usually not taught in traditional medicine.

creative arts therapists: Health care professionals who apply dance, art, music, drama, and poetry as treatment interventions for individuals with emotional, cognitive, and physical disorders. Most creative arts therapists have graduate degrees and require registration and certification from a professional association.

depression: A mood disorder that causes the individual to feel hopeless and sad, to lack energy, and to have problems eating and sleeping.

developmental disability: According to the Centers for Disease Control and Prevention, "Developmental disabilities are a group of conditions due to an impairment in physical, learning, language, or behavior areas. These conditions begin during the developmental period, may impact day-to-day functioning, and usually last throughout a person's lifetime." Examples of a developmental disability include autism, cerebral palsy, and Down syndrome.

disability: A functional impairment due to cognitive, motor, emotional, or sensory disorder that interferes with the ability to do the everyday tasks of living.

Down syndrome: A genetic disorder that causes mild, moderate, or severe intellectual disability.

ergonomics: The science and technology of fitting and adapting the environment to increase human function and to prevent work injuries.

group therapy: An intervention to help individuals to gain insight into their own problems by obtaining support and encouragement from the therapist and other members of the group.

habilitation: The intervention process of helping individuals, such as those with developmental disabilities, gain cognitive, sensory, and motor skills.

handicap: The inability to perform functional skills because of environmental barriers or disabilities.

hemiplegia: A paralysis of one side of the body, frequently occurring after a stroke.

instrumental activities of daily living: Everyday tasks that involve money management, public transportation use, home management (such as cleaning, cooking, and baking), safety precautions in the home, and leisure activities.

joint protection: Use of assistive devices, such as splints or slings, and procedures to minimize the stress and wear and tear on joints.

kinesthesia: Ability to sense the position in space and the direction of joint movements.

learning disability or disorder: Difficulty in learning academic subjects in a classroom setting. Special education is prescribed.

manual therapy: Interventions or protocols to increase hand movements and coordination, reduce edema, and alleviate pain.

Medicaid: A federally funded program administered by states to provide medical care for low-income individuals.

medical model: Traditional Western medicine treatment that is based on prevention, etiology, diagnosis, pharmaceutical prescriptions, surgery, and hospital care.

Medicare: A federally funded mandate to provide health insurance for people older than 65 years of age.

multiple sclerosis: A disease of the nervous system causing muscle weakness, problems with walking, visual disturbances, and disordered coordination.

occupational therapy: According to the American Occupational Therapy Association, "Occupational therapy is the only profession that helps people across the lifespan to do the things they want and need to do through the therapeutic use of daily activities (occupations). Occupational therapy practitioners enable people of all ages to live life to its fullest by helping them promote health, and prevent—or live better with—injury, illness, or disability."

orthotics: Devices, such as braces or splints, to compensate for an injury or to prevent further injury.

osteoarthritis: A chronic disease usually occurring in older people that affects the joints, such as the knees, hips, hands, and feet. It reduces movements and causes pain.

pain management: Interventions that include pharmaceutical and non-pharmaceutical procedures, such as opioids and other drugs, massage, acupuncture, exercise, chiropractic approaches, and surgery.

paraplegia: Paralysis of the legs usually caused by an injury.

Parkinson's disease: A chronic progressive disease of the central nervous system that causes hand tremors, incoordination, slurred speech, and cognitive disabilities.

physical agent modalities: Physical agents, such as heat, cold, ultrasound, vibration, and massage.

physical therapist: A health and rehabilitation professional who concentrates on improving the patient's mobility, relieving pain, and increasing strength, for example, through therapeutic exercise, patient education, electrical modalities, massage, and hydrotherapy. The entry-level for practice is a doctorate in physical therapy.

post-traumatic stress disorder: Usually occurs after a disturbing experience, such as in war, a car accident, rape, or other life-threatening event. Symptoms include depression, drug addictions, anxiety, hopelessness, insomnia, and eating disorders.

progressive muscle relaxation: A technique to help the patient relax through systematically flexing and relaxing the muscles of the body.

relaxation therapy: A technique using meditation to help the patient deal with stress and anxiety.

rheumatoid arthritis: A chronic systemic disease that causes inflammation to the joints with resulting pain and limitations in performing everyday movements.

schizophrenia: A severe psychiatric disorder in which patients experience hallucinations, delusions, and distorted thinking.

sensory integration: A theoretical framework in occupational therapy. It refers to the use of sensory stimulation and sensory feedback in helping a child, or sometimes an adult, integrate sensory stimuli. It includes vestibular stimulation, balance activities, and bilateral motor coordination activities.

speech-language pathologist: A health and rehabilitation professional who evaluates and treats individuals with communication disorders resulting from stroke, brain injury, hearing loss, developmental delay, Parkinson's disease, a cleft palate, or autism, and also swallowing problems. A master's degree is required for licensure and practice.

spinal cord injury: An injury to the spinal cord resulting in either weakness or paralysis in movements, such as inability to walk or, in cases of high-level injuries, an inability to use one's arms. Many spinal cord injuries are the result of car accidents or diving in a shallow pool.

stress management: An intervention program that attempts to help the patient reduce distress through relaxation techniques, music, yoga, exercise, social support, abdominal breathing, and personal counseling.

stroke rehabilitation: A combined effort by occupational therapy, physical therapy, speech pathology, audiology, and medical personnel to restore function in an individual who has experienced a stroke.

therapeutic activities: Purposeful and meaningful interventions that prevent disability and restore function in individuals with disabilities.

therapeutic exercise: Prescribed by a therapist, purposeful exercise such as aerobic exercise (e.g., running), aquatic activity, or weight-lifting.

traumatic brain injury: Injury to the brain causing cognitive disability.

work conditioning or work hardening: A comprehensive program to help the injured worker return to a job or to recommend accommodations in the work environment to help the injured worker to be able to do the job. The return-to-work program includes muscle-strengthening and simulated work samples to evaluate the person's ability to return to work.

Bibliography

America's Navy. (n.d.). Occupational therapy careers. Retrieved from https://www.navy.com/careers/occupational-therapy

American Occupational Therapy Association Representative Assembly 4/14/11 (Agenda A13, Charge 18)

American Occupational Therapy Association. (n.d.). Retrieved from https://www.aota.org/

American Occupational Therapy Association. (2015). *Occupational therapy code of ethics*. Bethesda, MD: Author.

American Occupational Therapy Association. (2015). *Salary & workforce survey*. Bethesda, MD: AOTA Press.

American Occupational Therapy Association. (n.d.). What is occupational therapy? Retrieved from https://www.aota.org/Conference-Events/OTMonth/what-is-OT.aspx

Andersen, L. T., & Reed, K. L. (2017). *The history of occupational thearpy: The first century.* Thorofare, NJ: SLACK Incorporated.

Association of Schools Advancing Health Professions. (2015, October 27). What is allied health? Retrieved from https://www.asahp.org/what-is

Barton, G. E. (1914). A view of invalid occupation. *Trained Nurse and Hospital Review, 52*(6), 327-330.

Bureau of Labor Statistics, U. S. Department of Labor. (2020, September 28). *Occupational outlook handbook: Occupational therapy assistants and aides.* Retrieved October 15, 2020, from https://www.bls.gov/ooh/healthcare/occupational-therapists.htm

Centers for Disease Control and Prevention. (2019, September 26). Facts about developmental disorders. Retrieved from https://www.cdc.gov/ncbddd/developmentaldisabilities/facts.html

CollegeScholarships.com. (n.d.). Occupational therapy scholarships. Retreived from https://www.collegescholarships.com/major-degree/occupational-therapy-scholarships

CostHelper Education. (n.d.). Becoming an occupational therapist cost. Retrieved from https://www.education.costhelper.com/occupational-therapist.html

Doyle, A. (2019, December 20). Types of employee benefits and perks. Retrieved January 17, 2019, from https://www.thebalancecareers.com/types-of-employee-benefits-and-perks-2060433#:~:text=These%20perks%2C%20also%20known%20as,work%3B%20retirement%20and%20pension%20plan

Early Childhood Technical Assistance Center. (n.d.). Federal definitions of assistive technology. Retrieved from https://www.ectacenter.org/topics/atech/definitions.asp

GoCoastGuard.com. (n.d.). Clinical and rehabilitation therapist. Retrieved from https://www.gocoastguard.com/active-duty-careers/officer-opportunities/programs/clinical-and-rehabilitation-therapist

McNary, H. (1954). The scope of occupational therapy. In H. Willard and C. Spackman (Eds.). Principles of occupational therapy, 2nd edition (pp.11-23). J. B. Lippincott: Philadelphia, PA.

National Board for Certification in Occupational Therapy. (n.d.). Retrieved from https://www.nbcot.org

National Board for Certification in Occupational Therapy. (2018). *Candidate/Certificant Code of Conduct.* Available online at www.nbcot.org

National Board for Certification in Occupational Therapy. (2020). *Certification exam handbook.* Retrieved from https://www.nbcot.org/-/media/NBCOT/PDFs/Cert_Exam_Handbook.ashx

O-Net OnLine. (2020, August 18). *Summary report for: 31-2011.00—occupational therapy assistants.* Retrieved February 19, 2020, from https://www.onetonline.org/link/summary/31-2011.00

PayScale. (n.d.). Average Certified Occupational Therapy Assistant (COTA) hourly pay. Retrieved from https://www.payscale.com/research/US/Job=Certified_Occupational_Therapy_Assistant_(COTA)/Hourly_Rate

Reed, K. L. (2014). Table of contents. In: *Quick Reference to Occupational Therapy.* Austin, TX: ProEd.

Top Occupational Therapy Schools. (n.d.). Differences between occupational therapists and occupational therapy assistants. Retrieved from https://www.topoccupationaltherapyschool.com/ot-vs-ota-difference/

Top Occupational Therapy Schools. (n.d.). Scholarships and grants for occupational therapists. Retrieved from https://www.topoccupationaltherapyschool.com/scholarships-grants-occupational-therapists/

Tracy, S. E. (1910). *Studies in invalid occupation: A manual for nurses and attendants.* Boston, MA: Whitcomb & Barrows.

U. S. Air Force. (n.d.). Occupational therapist. Retrieved from https://www.airforce.com/careers/detail/occupational-therapist

U. S. Army. (n.d.). Careers and jobs: Medical specialist corps. Retrieved from https://www.goarmy.com/careers-and-jobs/amedd-categories/medical-specialist-corps-jobs.html?AR=both&selectCategory=medical-corps-jobs

U. S. Army. (n.d.). Careers and jobs: Occupational therapist (65A). Retrieved from https://www.goarmy.com/careers-and-jobs/amedd-categories/medical-specialist-corps-jobs/occupational-therapist.html

U. S. Army. (n.d.). Partnership for youth success. Retrieved from https://www.armypays.com

U. S. Bureau of Labor Statistics. (n.d.). Occupational outlook handbook. Retrieved from https://www.bls.gov/ooh/

U. S. Department of Education. (2008, February 26). Recognition of foreign qualifications. Retrieved from https://www.ed.gov/about/offices/list/ous/international/usnei/us/edlite-visitus-forrecog.html

Wisconsin Occupational Therapy Association. (n.d.). Retrieved from https://www.wota.net

World Federation of Occupational Therapists. (n.d.). Retrieved from https://www.wfot.org

INDEX

Printed in the United States
by Baker & Taylor Publisher Services